The Sustained Fitness Transformation

Trey Patterson

The Sustained Fitness Transformation
Copyright © 2024 by Trey Patterson

Published in Dallas, Texas, by Let's Go! Press

All rights reserved. No part of this publication may be reproduced, stored in a retrieval system, or transmitted in any form or by any means—electronic, mechanical, photocopy, recording, or any other—except for brief quotations in critical reviews or articles, without the prior permission of the publisher.

Unless otherwise stated, all Scripture quotations are taken from the Holy Bible, New International Version®, NIV®. Copyright © 1973, 1978, 1984, 2011 by Biblica, Inc.® Used by permission. All rights reserved worldwide.

Scripture quotations marked (NKJV) are taken from New King James Version®. Copyright © 1982 by Thomas Nelson. Used by permission. All rights reserved.

ISBN 979-8-9913938-0-5 (paperback)

Library of Congress Control Number: 2024917805

Printed in The United States
10 9 8 7 6 5 4 3 2 1

Contents

Part I
Train With Trey- Introduction to The Sustained Fitness Transformation

Chapter 1: Meet Your Trainer...1

Chapter 2: Prepare for Growth..11

Chapter 3: Dismantle Diet Culture...17

Trey's 4-Step Evolution of Change

Chapter 4: The Power of the Mind...27

Chapter 5: Turn Thoughts into Actions..37

Chapter 6: Create a Great Outcome..47

Trey's Process for Sustained Transformation

Chapter 7: Enjoy The Process...59

Chapter 8: Reclaim Your Environment..69

Chapter 9: The Life of Discipline...77

Chapter 10: You're a Diamond...89

Mentalities and Mindsets for Your Motivation

Chapter 11: Victor/Champion Mentality...97

Chapter 12: Humble/Confident/Rich Mentality..........................105

Chapter 13: Progress and Investment Mindset............................113

Part II
Trey's Triad of Success

Chapter 14: The Triad of Success Explained................................121

Chapter 15: The Complexity of Diet...131

Chapter 16: The Gut...143

Chapter 17: Sugar..153

Chapter 18: Hormones..163

The Society Roadblocks to Success

Chapter 19: The Great Distractions..177

Chapter 20: Inactivity and Over-Accessibility................................189

Chapter 21: Validation and Manipulation.......................................199

Your Goals

Chapter 22: Small Steps, Distance Traveled...................................213

Chapter 23: Make Creative Goals..221

Chapter 24: It's Action Time...231

Chapter 25: The Life of Purpose..237

Acknowledgements...249

Stay Connected..251

Citations..252

-Chapter 1-
Meet Your Trainer

"Wow... I remember you... I didn't even recognize you... I'm so proud of how much you've changed." -Hugh Jones, former principal of Hebron High School

As a troubled teenager, at just 12 years of age, I fell into drug and alcohol addiction. I was a teenager with an identity crisis. Like a lot of teenagers, I had trouble discovering who I was, what I wanted to be, who I fit in with, and I struggled making friends. By the age of 15, after multiple school expulsions, and getting in trouble with the law, I had a rock-bottom experience in a jail cell and began my quest for personal change. I spent the next two and a half weeks in a jail cell reflecting on life and how to change my life. With multiple offenses on my record as a teenager, I knew that I could not continue with my actions or I'd either end up dead or in prison before I even graduated high school. The trajectory of my life wasn't positive.

After spending two and a half weeks in a jail cell, which felt like hell, I was ready to change my behavior. In the pursuit of change, and being court ordered, at 15 years of age I started attending

Alcoholics Anonymous (AA) meetings. To answer your question, yes, I was the youngest person in every AA meeting I ever attended. After getting released from jail, it became official, I had been expelled from my high school. Because of the expulsion, I was then sentenced to eight months in a juvenile detention military school. Military school was my only chance to be re-admitted to the high school that I had been previously expelled from. I was completely cut off from my old environment. New school, new classmates, and my parents had even moved into a new house.

"Behavior adjustment" was the goal of my marine core drill instructors at military school. Upon entry into the school, they broke me down and made me cry, as this was part of their agenda to rebuild us. I thought I was bad. Here I am, on day one, crying while five drill instructors made me hold a plank for 20-30 minutes screaming in my face telling me how weak and worthless I am. This was a common practice anytime they felt like I needed correction. I had to learn to enjoy the pain. I even told one of my drill sergeants that I wanted to change my life, and I'd be open to whatever he could offer me. In desperation to change my life, I embraced the screams in my face, I took pride in ironing my military fatigues, and I enjoyed showing my sergeants how good I was at polishing my boots. I embraced all the disciplines that I was required to develop. And I absolutely loved decimating all of my classmates in physical training by running the fastest mile, beating them in the pushup challenge, and always winning in the obstacle course. After eight months, and at 16 years of age, I left the school as the highest ranking corporal. That's something to make your mother proud of right?

While many around me weren't privileged, I had an amazing upbringing. I had two parents who loved me unconditionally and fought to give me the best life that they could give me. Yet from a very young age, I still struggled with extreme depression, suicidal thoughts, and an addictive personality that brought an insurmountable amount of destruction. After exiting military school, I wanted all the more to become someone so dramatically different than who I used to be. I got active in church. I had a radical encounter with a real God- not a religion. I gave my life to Jesus Christ. I became a born-again Christian, on fire for God, and spent most of my free time pursuing God. Most of my old friends thought I'd lost my mind and wanted nothing to do with me, which was perfectly fine. Salvation would have it that I would be cut off from my old friends and would eventually form new friends that would build me up and help me to become the better version of me.

At 17 years of age, I got involved in a group called Overcomers, which was a Christ-based 12-step program, similar to AA. The leader of the group was a woman by the name of Cynthia Corder. In every single group meeting that we had, we took time to verbally make a declaration of who we are in Christ and how we are overcomers. These declarations were inspired by two Bible verses. The first one is Romans 12:2a, "Do not conform to the pattern of this world, but be transformed by the renewing of your mind." The second verse, Proverbs 23:7a (NKJV) states: "For as he thinks in his heart, so is he." The power of declaration is a concept that was even practiced by Andrew Carnegie. It's documented that Andrew Carnegie looked at himself in the mirror every day and declared that one day he was going to become the richest man in the world. He became the very person that seemed so unrealistic for him to become. Andrew Carnegie one day became the richest man in the world. The message of self-declaration, the shifting of thoughts, and the understanding of identity became a major pillar in my life of change and transformation. This message on the power of identity became so deeply rooted within me, so much so, that every morning and night for the next year I would proclaim destiny and good things over myself. "One day I'm going to change the entire world." I believed it. The world began to appear small to me and reaching the entire world seemed like not just a possibility, but a capability. I was undergoing an identity change.

My senior year of high school, at 18 years of age, I was invited by one of my teachers to speak in front of my fellow high school classmates at an FCA (Fellowship of Christian Athletes) meeting and share my story. I remember the day like it was yesterday, and it would become a memory that I'd never forget. As I stood up to speak in front of the 30-40 classmates, in came walking the principal of my high school. My principal, Hugh Jones, was the head principal of Hebron High School from the time I was a rambunctious freshman. I shared my story of transformation, from being a destructive teenager to a born-again Christian. Afterward, Mr. Jones approached me and said, "Wow... I remember you... I didn't even recognize you... I'm so proud of how much you've changed." It was the first time in my life that I had a true realization of how much I had changed. In just a three year period, I had become unrecognizable!

There was one chief factor that lead to my dramatic three year transformation. I had the will and desire to change my life. It was the will and the determination to hold onto the disciplines created at military school. It was the will and the determination to follow God. It wasn't just "I want" to change my life, it was "I must" change my life. I realized that anything in life was possible, as long as I want it bad enough.

By the age of 18, I became wildly optimistic and developed a deep love and an empathy for those struggling with my previous struggles of addiction and depression. During this time, I was introduced to a woman named Kim Smith who was the founder of a non-profit called Journey to Dream. Little did I know that over the next six years, from the age of 18-24, I would become an established motivational speaker through Journey to Dream as well as a couple of other drug awareness organizations and church groups. Over those six years, I would have the opportunity to speak to over 60,000 students throughout the Dallas Fort Worth metroplex. I would share my story of hope and transformation to middle schoolers and high schoolers on a regular basis, and I would talk about the power of the mind and self belief. The high that I would experience from speaking in front of a thousand kids in a single day, is unparalleled to any high I've ever received from any drug prior. I came to realize at this point in my life that I loved being a positive influence on others. It wasn't just a passion of mine; it became my purpose. I loved the feeling of walking away knowing that I changed someone else's life. My day was always made when a student would walk up to me anywhere, whether it was a shopping mall, restaurant, or gas station, because they remembered me speaking at their school and would share how much my speech impacted them. My greatest passion became influencing behavior, and this passion would follow me into the next several chapters of my life.

  During this time in my life, when I was 20 years old, I got bit by the fitness bug. I can honestly say that fitness became an obsession. I couldn't wait to get out of class so that I could go workout, and a large percentage of my free time was dedicated to studying anything fitness related. Through a transformed mind, came a transformed body. After graduating from Dallas Baptist University with a degree in Communications, I got pulled into the fitness industry by a man named Tim McComsey. He had his own fitness business, was a published fitness model, and a man I view as a mentor even to this day. Following in his footsteps, I started competing in what is arguably the most difficult sport in the world, bodybuilding. A sport that not only challenges your physical limits, but challenges your mental grit and produces strict discipline. Over my competition history, I would place at some of the most competitive shows in Texas, including Mr. Europa. The body will only achieve what the mind believes. With a calling as a motivational speaker and a passion for fitness, I then became a group fitness instructor and spent the next five years working full time for one the largest boutique fitness chains in DFW. There I trained 500+ people on a weekly basis motivating them to push past what they *think* their limitations are. During this time in my life, I met and fell in love with Monica Bustamante and today we are happily married. In February of 2020, a few months after getting married, I resigned from my position at the boutique gym. It was bittersweet as I had built many friendships and connections, yet I felt a freedom to conquer greater territories. Big things were in store… Or were they?

    During my transition to another fitness chain, Covid-19 struck. The fitness industry completely shut down. I had no job. No income coming in. I was devastated. I was left with uncertainty and only enough finances to get me through a couple of months. Desperate for work, I started selling $10 online workouts and offering extremely inexpensive personal training sessions just to make enough money to pay my basic bills. In just 1 month, I went from training 500 people on a weekly basis, to attempting to private message almost everyone I knew to try and support me as a personal trainer by buying my $10 online workouts. Prior to Covid, in my mind, I was Mr. Popular as I had trained tens of thousands of people throughout DFW. One month into Covid, I was in quarantine, isolated, doing personal training for a few people in my apartment garage basement, constantly having to move for cars driving by. And I was doing this level of training for half the price of what I was getting paid prior to Covid. I was humbled. "Is this my new norm?" Begging people to train them and doing it for half of what I was making prior to Covid?

It was a stark contrast to go from training 500 people on a weekly basis, to now training a few people in my parking garage basement, I felt like I wasn't making a significant difference. I always wanted to be that world changer, but it felt like my dreams were slipping away from me. I had to change my perspective and focus on the positive. Not everything is good, but you can find some good in everything. The first few months of Covid were the best months of my life in terms of growth. I was forced into a position where I needed to grow. Forced out of my nest of comfort, I needed to learn how to spread my own wings and fly. Most of my free time was spent on self-education. I started learning about investments and financial planning. While I was making enough money at the start of Covid just to get by, I was forced to cut out several luxuries that I was previously accustomed to. The humility that I experienced due to Covid was foundational to my growth. Out of the positive perspective, came a life promotion. Little did I know, I was in the process of forming my first business.

I made the decision that I wanted to be the best personal trainer to all my clients. I started studying more about health and fitness, and even pursued a couple more training certifications to increase my knowledge and value in the fitness industry. Through Covid quarantine, I continued personal training and online workouts. Within the first four months of Covid, I had a full schedule of clients. In June of 2020, the boutique fitness gym that was going to hire me prior to Covid offered me a job, which I decided to turn down. My business was moving forward, and without question, I wanted to remain committed to the clients that I had gained. Once gyms started reopening four months after quarantine started, I began doing outdoor group fitness classes at Vitruvian Park in Addison, Texas. I coached these classes together with a buddy of mine named Pedram Zaff. We wanted to create a safe Covid-friendly environment. The group classes saw a lot of growth during the summer of 2020, so much so that we actually got media attention on a couple of occasions, being featured on Good Morning Texas discussing the new era of fitness post-Covid. The process of starting my own business wasn't easy, but it sure was rewarding. I didn't just go through the process; I grew through it.

As a new fresh fire had arisen inside of me, I had officially formed my first business offering personal and group fitness training. The start of Covid marks the day that I officially became self-employed. The job struggle that I faced at the beginning of Covid became a blessing in disguise. Diligence is always rewarded. For the next several years, I would offer personal training and group classes to clients. I jokingly tell my friends and loved ones all the time that I'm unemployed and haven't had a job in years. They say that when you love what you do, you'll never work a day in your life. With a heightened passion for fitness and seeing my clients experiencing transformation, I became a certified Health and Wellness Coach. I've always had a deep desire to understand patterns of behaviors and incorporate health and wellness coaching into my training style. The year 2024 marks ten years of being full-time in the fitness industry. With the fire burning stronger than ever before, I want to help you become the healthiest, fittest version of you that you can be! I want to help unlock the potential within you!

How to Read This Book

The first half of this book (Chapters 1-13) is dedicated to the human mentality and how to create the transformation of the mind. Let's destroy the ideals of diet culture! Let's discover the 4-Step Evolution of Change! Let's take the journey of success in the process! Let's embrace the mentalities of success! The second half of this book (Chapters 14-25) is dedicated to practicality and how to achieve your physical transformation. Together we will discover the Triad of Success! Let's identify the societal roadblocks of success! Let's create goals and action plans to promote results! Scattered throughout this book, I have emboldened key points or thoughts that I believe need emphasis. And if you are looking for a quick pick-me-up motivational speech, at the end of several of the chapters, I have placed a short section entitled "Motivation for You." It's time to challenge all that we previously knew! It's time to go on the quest of discovery! It's time to unleash the power within you! This is *The Sustained Fitness Transformation!*

Sustained

Sustained: "kept in process or continued over time; continuous." -Dictionary.com

Fitness

Fitness: "the condition of being physically fit and healthy. The quality of being suitable to fulfill a particular role or task." -Oxford languages

Transformation

Transformation: "a complete change in the appearance or character of something or someone, especially so that the thing or person is improved." -Cambridge Dictionary

-Chapter 2-
Prepare for Growth

"Change is inevitable, but growth is a decision!"
-Trey Patterson

Before we get into the meat of the book, there are a few more terms that I would like to define as I will be using them frequently.

Health: "the condition of being sound in body, mind, or spirit. Especially: freedom from physical disease or pain." -Merriam-Webster

Process: "a series of actions or steps taken in order to achieve a particular end." -Oxford Languages

Exercise: "activity requiring physical effort, carried out to sustain or improve health and fitness." -Oxford Languages

Success: "the achieving of the results wanted or hoped for. Something that achieves positive results." -Cambridge Dictionary

Change: "make (someone or something) different; alter or modify. the act or instance of making or becoming different." -Oxford Languages

Joseph Campbell said, "We must be willing to let go of the life we've planned, as to have the life that is waiting for us."

You've got to be willing to let go of the life that you "want," in order to obtain the life that you deserve. What if I told you that in one year from now, you could one hundred percent change your life- mind, body, and soul? In one year from now, almost everything can change for the better. In one year you can be more successful, by whatever definition that is to you. You can be happier. You can physically feel better. You can have a better physique. Honest question, would you do whatever it takes to get there? It requires "out with the old, in with the new." Unfortunately it can be hard to lay down the old to make room for the new. Most people are willing to put one foot forward, but many keep one foot back. Without continuous efforts to step forward, there is no movement or change.

I'm going to paint a picture for you. The front foot symbolizes your future and the back foot symbolizes your past. The back foot represents comfort. The back foot represents security. The back foot is the place where you previously were. It's where you were 10 years ago, 5 years ago, 2 years ago, 3 months ago. It's the job you've been stagnant at for five years where you haven't had much recent development. The back foot is that relationship, friend, or romance that hasn't produced much positive in your life, but you've stayed there out of comfort. Your front foot symbolizes greater success, transformation, and change. The front foot symbolizes the vision and belief of what is obtainable. The new territory you can conquer. The greater successes you can step into. I believe the main reason people are afraid to step forward, or create movement, is because of a bad experience with a past failure. They've tripped along the way. There is nothing more crippling and destructive than fear. **Fear kills more dreams than failure ever will.**

Today, in this exact moment, you are the smartest that you've ever been. You are the strongest that you have ever been. You are the wisest that you have ever been. You have more experience and you have more knowledge than you've ever had. Because of this, **the odds of success are in your favor.** If you experienced a measure of success, dating back to 5 years ago, imagine if you went out with the old and in with the new. You are almost guaranteed to reach higher heights! Maybe you've had a boss instill the idea within you, "this is as good as it's going to get for you!" First off, a true leader will never try to minimize your potential. If you were qualified for your position 5 years ago, today, you are overqualified for that same position. Think of how much wisdom you've developed over the past 5 years, 2 years, or even 6 months. It doesn't matter if you've had a lot of screw ups or mess ups along the way, you have significantly increased in knowledge. There is no such thing as wasted time. Even if you think that you are behind where you are supposed to be, you've learned through life's processes. Don't compare yourself to someone else. They are running a different race and on a different timeline. You can accomplish more in the next five years than someone else can accomplish in their entire lifetime. The only thing holding you back is your back foot!

The odds are in your favor! Boldness and bravery are needed to step out and try something you've never tried before. The worst thing that can happen if you don't succeed is that you will fall right back to where you were. The time is right for you to lift that back foot and start moving forward. It's time to create movement. Falling is acceptable. Clawing is acceptable. Crawling is acceptable. But halting is not.

Transformation starts with your thoughts when you tell yourself that you can. One year from now, you can completely change your life for the better, but it does require out with the old and in with the new. It requires a daily lifting of that back foot and stepping toward your future. Life is not about coasting on a previous victory. It's about going from victory to victory.

Your transformation starts here!

Having the right mentalities and mindsets is a crucial part of your success in your transformation journey. Further along, we will discuss what I believe to be the most important mentalities and mindsets to usher in greater success. There is one mindset that I'd like to address before we proceed, as I believe it is foundational to your success. Growth mindset.

Growth Mindset

There is a tale of two identical twin boys. Their father was an alcoholic. As the twins grew older, they parted ways. Son A followed in his father's footsteps and became an alcoholic and ended up homeless. He had determined that he was supposed to be an alcoholic because it was in the cards. "I was destined to be an alcoholic." Son B became a very successful businessman and had determined that he would never drink alcohol. He was able to learn a lesson from his father and never even tried drinking alcohol. "I was destined for something greater than being an alcoholic." He believed in a greater opportunity. What was the fundamental difference between the two sons? One had a fixed mindset, the other had a growth mindset.

In order to further understand what growth mindset is, let's explore what fixed mindset is. A fixed mindset believes that circumstances, skills, experience, etc. are unchangeable. Fixed mindset is a "so be it" mindset or an "it is what it is" mindset. It also doesn't see much value in personal growth. "Why make effort to improve or grow because ultimately it doesn't matter?" A fixed mindset will keep you trapped in your current position. If you don't see the value in personal growth, it will be very difficult to accomplish greater things and it will be very difficult to create a profound change in your own life. If you want to become the smartest version of you, if you want to become the healthiest version of you, if you want to become the best version of you, it comes through a growth mindset. It all starts with seeing the value in personal growth.

I couldn't find statistics on how many people read at least one book per year, but I can imagine that it's substantially less than 50 percent. And of those that do read, it's probably substantially less than ten books per year. I was able to find a statistic on how many books the average CEO reads. While it may seem like a shock, the average CEO reads over 50 books per year. There is one fundamental difference between the average person and the CEO. Growth mindset. Growth mindset always has a curiosity, it always asks questions, it always seeks knowledge. It's the foundation of learning. The CEO didn't fall into a high position, they grew into it!

I've heard many motivational speakers talk about striving to become one percent better everyday, but none have addressed how you accomplish that. The way you become one percent better everyday is by waking up everyday and being intentional about seeking knowledge, seeking opportunity, and seeking growth.

"Improving by just one percent isn't notable (and sometimes it isn't even noticeable). But it can be just as meaningful, especially in the long run." -James Clear.

If you become one percent better everyday, you'll become over 37 times better after ten years! To say that someone will become "better" is an objective statement, but this is to paint the picture that improvement compounds over time. With a growth mindset, you can accomplish more in one year than someone else can accomplish in ten years. In fact, you can accomplish more in one year than some will accomplish in an entire lifetime.

Your greatest measure of growth does not come when things are going easy for you. Your greatest measure of growth comes in the times when you feel the pressures of life. Challenges, setbacks, and failures are inevitable. A growth mindset sees a challenge, setback, or even a failure as an opportunity. Don't be afraid of failing. You just need to fail forward. Just put one foot in front of the other and keep moving forward. Through everything that is inevitable, there is opportunity. As stated in my bio, not everything that happens is going to be good, but you can find some good in everything. **Change is inevitable but growth is a decision.** Your greatest growth comes from intention. Don't wake up and say, I'm going to try and make it through another day. Wake up and say I'm going to make an effort to learn through another day. Don't just go through your day, grow through your day.

Always strive to challenge old belief systems. Fixed mindset is a limiting belief system. Growth mindset seeks to expand the belief system. Knowledge is always changing and evolving, so strive to learn new knowledge. You have two options today; you can either step forward into growth, or you can step backward into comfort. You can either step forward into growth, or you can step backward into complacency. **It's okay to be content, but it's never okay to be complacent.** Every mindset is a decision, so choose a growth mindset!

-Chapter 3-
Dismantle Diet Culture

"The short-term perception of change and transformation that diet culture promotes is the most destructive ideology toward true change and transformation."
-Trey Patterson

"Trey, can you get me to lose 30 pounds in three months?" Yes, it's possible. Truthfully my main concern as a fitness, health, and wellness coach isn't getting you to lose 30 pounds in three months but rather giving you the tools for a sustainable fitness transformation. **Transformation does not come through one month of hard work, it's a long commitment to destroying old habits to make way for new habits.** My goal is to set you up with lifelong success in your fitness journey.

Before I continue on the topic of transformation and discuss what I'm going to call The 4-Step Evolution of Change, there is an issue that needs to be addressed. "Diet Culture." Unfortunately, diet culture has given us the wrong illustration of what transformation looks like and creates a short-term perception of transformation that can lead to unhealthy behaviors and attitudes. **The short-term perception of change and transformation that diet culture promotes is the most destructive ideology toward true change and transformation.** We've become accustomed to the "Lose 10 pounds in 10 days with my workout plan." Or the before and after pics of "I lost 20 pounds in six weeks" or similar. While results are something to applaud and serve as a sense of accomplishment, it's time to restructure the ideological constructs of what transformation is. Transformation is a journey and a never-ending process.

Most get stuck on the fitness roller coaster. We jump on fad diets, we obtain results, then lose those results, and repeat. Can you lose 30 pounds in three months? Yes, it's possible. This is what I can tell you from experience with this transformation mindset through training thousands of clients. At least 95 percent of the time, after the three months are up, or whatever the short-term time allotment is, they'll drift back into their old patterns. In many cases, after jumping on a fad diet plan, they end up having a rebound where almost all of their hard work becomes lost. Diet culture creates a result-based mentality, not a long-term transformation mentality. It creates an outcome-based mentality, not a process-based mentality. **At an atomic level, when the transformation of a cell takes place, it can never rebound and return to its previous structure.** Transformation isn't just about physical results, it's the permanent change in DNA- mind, body, soul.

"Have you heard about the new diet?!?! I've been hearing that many are losing over ten pounds a month on this new diet and it's really easy!"

Fad Diets

Diet culture promotes a fad diet. A fad diet is a trendy weight loss plan that offers quick and dramatic results. Here are a few examples of fad diets that we've all heard about. One of the biggest ones is the Paleo Diet. The Paleo Diet, also referred to as the "caveman diet," promotes eating natural foods obtained from hunting and gathering. It's a higher protein diet consisting of lean meats, vegetables, nuts, and fruits. The goal is to eliminate all processed foods and unnatural sugars. Another common fad diet is the Keto Diet. The Keto Diet is a very unique diet. Most diets are "high protein, low carb diets" while the Keto Diet is a high fat, medium protein and low carb diet. When 80 percent of your diet consists of the fats, your body will flip into ketosis. Ketosis occurs when your body doesn't have enough carbs to convert to energy. Instead, it utilizes the fats for the energy. Of your three macronutrients (protein, carbs, fats), fats actually produce the most energy. So, when consuming high amounts of fats, you will not feel the "dieting lack of energy" even when in a caloric deficit. Another popular diet is the Atkins Diet. It's a diet still commonly used today, and it has been around since the 1970's. This diet is referred to as the original low carb diet. And because of its low carb nature, it encourages the restriction of many fruits, vegetables, and grains. And it highly encourages the consumption of meats (protein source) and fatty fish, yogurt, and dairy (fat sources).

So which one would I recommend? Drum roll…. None of them!

Why did I take the time to discuss fad diets, in particular, these fad diets? It's because there is key knowledge within these diets that we can learn from. Almost every fad diet is scientifically backed to be effective in delivering "results." Fad diets have been around for a long time, and not a single diet is one-size-fits-all. In fact, there is an unhealthy element to fad diets that needs to be addressed. Many of these fad diets encourage a caloric restriction and depletion of vital macronutrients that can actually lead to an even more unhealthy version of you.

  The new diet comes out, people start trying it, people start seeing results, and word shoots out about this new "effective" diet. Fad diets are effective at giving temporary results. But, there is one fundamental issue with these fad diets. It encourages you to go "on" a diet. On a psychological level, who wants to be on a diet? And, it's almost impossible to sustain a fad diet which is mainly because of the lack of enjoyment. Finding enjoyment in the process is possibly the largest contributor to success in your health and fitness journey. I have yet to meet anyone who has remained on the same diet for more than a couple of years. I've known a few people that have lost over 50 pounds within a year or two on the Keto Diet, but needed to stop because of health complications.

  The second reason why I do not recommend fad diets is because fad diets are business. Diet culture is promoted through the dieting industry. Scientists will create a new weight loss theory. That theory proves to be effective so now a "product" is created. "Lose 15 pounds in one month with our diet plan and supplements." Through marketing the product, a business is created. Sometimes the branding on these products is so good that it'll make you want to try it. The purpose of a business is to make money. It's important to understand that a lot of health, wellness, and nutritionist influencers on social media are selling the products that the companies pay them to sell. While some of the products that they sell truly are healthy, there is a secondary influence behind what they are selling- money! You're not getting sold the best product, you're getting sold the product that has the financial backing behind it. **And on a side note, it's important to understand that the dieting industry is trying to make you insecure, so that they can capitalize off of your insecurity.** They are trying to make you believe you are not good looking enough. They are trying to make you believe that you are not healthy enough. They are trying to make you believe that you need their product. It's sales.

Fad diets generally aren't healthy. Most advise that if you'd like to lose weight, you need to be on an extreme calorie deficit. I'm going to make a very bold and controversial statement, and it goes against everything that diet culture has taught us about dieting and weight loss. **Calorie restriction should never be the focus point of your weight loss journey.** Diet culture promotes the calorie restriction approach to weight loss. Calorie restriction is an outdated, ineffective, unhealthy, and a flawed approach to weight loss. The outcome is usually disastrous when the focus becomes calorie restriction. What happens with this approach is that people begin to decrease their calorie intake. They start seeing a weight reduction. "I must be doing something right!" Then they hit the plateau. What I've witnessed with this caloric restriction approach is that most of the time they end up decreasing their calories further, and it becomes a cycle. I've had multiple people approach me for personal training. "Trey, I can't seem to break through this plateau. I keep cutting my calorie intake and I'm currently only eating 900 calories per day and I still want to lose another 20 pounds." I've even had people approach me who have created such unhealthy patterns that they are on the verge of starvation from eating so few calories or eating only one meal per day. The calorie restriction model will promote and support an eating disorder. In fact, most of my clients that have an eating disorder, developed their eating disorder from this calorie deficit ideology.

The largest reason this approach is ineffective at helping the individual with a weight loss goal is because the metabolism will significantly slow down as less calories are consumed. Then what? You'll then be forced to consume less calories if you are to have the same weight loss benefit from this approach. This can cause a permanent negative effect on your metabolism and you can become extremely unhealthy in the process. It never ends well! When restricting calories, you might be depriving yourself of necessary macronutrients (fats, carbs, proteins), which support certain body functions. Meanwhile your body is not getting the fuel it needs. The lack of fuel is more damaging to the car than poor quality fuel. Of course some of the foods consumed on these fad diets might be healthier foods, but the elimination of vital macronutrients (fats, carbs, protein), on the health side, can create greater health issues than eating a surplus of junk food. Fad diets promote the deprivation of macronutrients. You can significantly increase your metabolism by eating more of the right foods. **It's not about eating less food; it's about eating the right food!** The more important question to ask is not how many calories, but which kind of calories?

A New Approach to Diet is Needed

If it's not about less food, but it's about the right foods, then what are the right foods? All of us have a general idea about what foods are healthy and what foods are not healthy. We know to eat our vegetables at dinner and stay away from fast food. Having the knowledge of what foods are best for your body type isn't a quick discovery. We do have great resources in place to help you discover the right foods for you. But even then, the body will change and health conditions will change making it impossible to discover the perfect diet. There is no one-size-fits-all diet as everyone's body responds differently to different foods. Everyone has different food sensitivities, food allergies, gluten sensitivities, and differing quality in produce and selection. In part two of this book, in the sub-section entitled "The Triad of Success," I'm going to share a few key resources to help you discover the right foods for you.

Everyone has different underlying medical conditions that affect food metabolism. For example, varying insulin sensitivities from person to person is going to affect how an individual converts certain foods into energy, especially in regards to the conversion of carbohydrate sources into energy. Insulin sensitivity is a topic that I will be discussing more in depth further in the book. I'll even make a challenge that eating a surplus of the right food can actually eliminate the medical issues that are causing adverse effects on the body such as weight gain. On a side note, another good resource is working with an experienced dietitian as they will help you understand foods and your body. A dietitian can provide you with many beneficial tests to help you discover the right foods for your body type. And a skilled dietitian can also help clients with eating behaviors, which for many is a key element to success in their dieting journey.

Diet culture promotes a result-based mentality which leads to unhealthy behaviors and attitudes. Through these unhealthy behaviors and attitudes, a roller coaster effect is created. Fast results, fast rebounds. It even causes you to be shameful of what you ate during the holidays and tells you it's time to diet on January 1st. Diet shaming is a struggle for many of us and dieting shaming will come from one of two sources, an outside source (other people) and your internal source (personal shaming). In fact, I'm going to teach you a little psychology trick to combat diet shaming. Rewire your mind not to label food as "good" or "bad." Rather, use the term "beneficial" or "non-beneficial." Labeling a food as a bad food suggests that you engaged in a wrongful behavior. As the term non-beneficial suggests, you ate a food that isn't going to add benefit toward you accomplishing your goals. If you are someone that struggles with the roller coaster effect and it's due to constant calorie restriction/binge eating cycles, I have another psychology trick for you. Change your mindset from "less food consumption" to "more nutrient dense food consumption." This mindset allows you to eat to your satisfaction. You're not restricting, you're enhancing. This mindset will help eliminate the restrict/binge cycle. Less is not always better. Remember this, not all calories are the same. But at the end of the day, stop shaming yourself. One meal isn't going to destroy all your hard-earned work.

Diet culture promotes the quick fix. To the diet pill generation- You may see the initial effects of a diet pill or diet medication, but again, it's something you cannot sustain. If it's a diuretic-based pill or medication you'll lose water weight which isn't true weight. You'll gain pretty much one hundred percent of it back the moment that you stop taking it, and in some cases, even more because of a rebound effect. Caffeine-based pills and medications? You may reap benefit from consuming caffeine to assist in weight loss, but in order to continue seeing results you need to constantly increase the dosage. This can lead to many bad health consequences. Caffeine is one of the most addictive drugs. When you stop taking caffeine, you will experience a crash of energy. Possibly the largest market of diet drugs is based upon those that suppress appetite. This will allow you to eat less unhealthy foods, right? Most of the time when someone comes off of a drug that suppresses appetite, they have a rebound with intense cravings.

We have become accustomed to the quick-fix culture. It's because we live in a fast-paced, microwave culture that we want the drug. Taking the drug may alleviate symptoms but it is ineffective at getting to the root of the issue. I do believe that the medical industry can add a lot of value in helping an individual achieve results especially if someone has an inhibiting medical condition, but it should never be the go-to solution. There is no magic, one-size-fits-all drug that doesn't come with potential adverse effects. The topic of inhibiting medical conditions is a topic that I'll be discussing in the sub-section of this book entitled "The Triad of Success."

Okay, let's take a deep breath. That was a lot of hard information and a tough pill to swallow, no pun intended. A new approach to our health and fitness journey is needed.

The key to success is in developing a lifestyle change that is formed from new habits. And you have to enjoy these new habits as this is the only way that it can be sustainable. What does it matter if you lose 30 pounds in three months, yet for the next 60 years of your life you still struggle with keeping off the weight or even simply remaining healthy for that matter? Fad diets or diet drugs may temporarily fix the issue of weight loss, but they do not fix the root of the issue of what's leading to the weight gain.

The transformation process is the long-term commitment to destroying old habits to make room for new habits. Think adjective, not noun. It is the ongoing process of change and development in our mind, body, and soul. Within the mind, it's the changing of our thoughts. Within the body, it's the physical changes that take place. Within the soul, it's the changing of passions, motivations, and emotions. The word change implies an outcome, while transformation implies a journey. If people start exercising with a goal of losing weight, after a month they may start to notice a physical change. If people continually see a physical change, if they are constantly working to improve their habits, if they are working to develop new mindsets, they are undergoing the process of transformation. In the same way that the cells in our body are always changing and replacing themselves, we are always transforming. I want to paint the picture of what transformation is. If I use the phrase "you can transform your life," I'm not referring to something outcome-based, I'm referring to a process. Now, changing your lifestyle does take work undeniably and sometimes the work is challenging. I'm not here to sell a quick fix. But on the flip side, I'm here to affirm that all the hard work is rewarding. My goal is to set you up with transformation!

-Chapter 4-
The Power of the Mind

*"You create your reality by what you believe.
You create your reality by what you think."*
-Trey Patterson

"It's not the movement on the clock that produces the newness of life. It is the movement in your mind. "Next year" isn't going to make you a new you. A new suit doesn't make you a new man. A new house doesn't make a new marriage. A new life comes from a new mind and a new way of looking at your life. You cannot step into the future and still think in your past. It's not what other people say about you that will bring you down, it's what you say about you." -T.D. Jakes.

Just how powerful is the mind?

Everything in our reality today started off as a thought. Every invention and every accomplishment started off as a belief. The invention of the plane was first invented in someone's mind. The creation of the internet was first created in someone's mind. Every advancement in our society was generated through the mind. A simple idea and visualization led to a creation. **You create your reality by what you believe. You create your reality by what you think.** If you want to create a new reality, you've got to create a new mind. The mind is central to all creation. The mind is central to your formation.

Healthy Mind, Healthy Life

At a physical level, your mind affects your health. A healthy mind, a healthy life. Psychosomatic illnesses are illnesses caused by poor mental states such as anxiety, depression, and stress that produce unhealthy physiological changes. Some of these include digestive issues, high blood pressure, headaches, fatigue, dizziness, and muscle aches. If these unhealthy physiological changes aren't addressed, they can progress into severe illness and even have fatal consequences. Medically speaking, the root cause of many severe illnesses is a poor mental state.

Somatic symptom disorder is an extreme focus on a physical symptom that can cause emotional distress and problems functioning. The most common type of somatic symptom disorder that many of us are familiar with is hypochondria which is an intense fear of a greater illness. Another very common type of somatic symptom disorder is body dysmorphia. Body dysmorphia is an obsessive focus on a perceived flaw. It is becoming more common in our society. This causes anxiety or emotional distress which can lead to unhealthy physiological changes. Medically speaking, the intense fear of developing illness can lead to illness. The extreme anxiety and emotional distress from body dysmorphia can negatively affect your health.

While doctors can prescribe medicines that alleviate the symptoms such as anti-depressants for depression and anti-anxiety meds for anxiety, the actual treatment for somatic symptom disorder is cognitive behavior therapy. Cognitive behavior therapy is a psychological therapy that helps you become aware of inaccurate or negative thinking and respond in a positive and more effective way. In its simplicity, the solution is positive meditation and positive mind renewal. Your thoughts have a direct correlation to your health.

The Power of Suggestion

If your thought processes have that strong of an impact on your life, then it's extremely important for us to guard our minds. Every day, we are introduced to different suggestions through the people around us, music, movies, etc. These suggestions have a subliminal effect on our thought processes. The psychology definition of the word "suggestion" according to the Macmillan Dictionary is "the action of influencing someone to make a mental connection between one thing and another."

Let's use a child watching a horror movie about sharks as an illustration of the power of suggestion. A child is extremely susceptible to suggestion because they are in a stage of development. Movies and television are two of the most powerful sources of suggestion because they create focus on not just imagery but sounds as well. And, movies and television stimulate emotions which will make an individual even more susceptible to suggestion. A child watching a horror movie about sharks can create a lifelong fear of the deep sea. In a graphic scene of a human being killed by a shark, that scene will produce powerful emotions such as fear, sadness, anger, etc. It can create a mental connection between the deep sea and sharks, and even as that child grows older, they may still have a fear of the deep sea and sharks. While children have a greater measure of susceptibility, adults are susceptible as well to suggestions. Suggestion impacts belief. Belief impacts destiny. If you want to change your destiny, surround yourself with positive suggestions through the movies you watch, the people you surround yourself with, and the music you listen to.

The main tool that psychologists use to help with negative suggestion impact is image visualization. For example, if you have a fear of the deep sea, a psychologist might suggest, "submerse yourself in a pool and visualize you are submersing yourself into the deep sea." Simple visualizations can help an individual overcome fears. Many athletes hire psychologists to help them with athletic performance. They use a tactic called guided imagery to promote image visualization. An example can be a psychologist guiding a basketball player through making a free throw. "Close your eyes. Now feel the ball gripped between your fingers. Bring the ball up to your chest and shoot the ball. Swoosh. Did you hear the swoosh?" It seems silly, but it is a tactic used by many professional athletes. It's a form of meditation that can help with performance.

There are many sports where image visualization is central to the sport. Golf is a great example. A golfer who is in tune with their clubs and their swing will take a few practice swings before they hit the ball. They'll practice the swing and visualize hitting the ball. Just through a practice swing, they know exactly how the ball will be released from the club. Once they practice the swing and discover the right club and intensity to hit the ball, they will then step up to hit the ball in the same manner that they visualized it being hit in their practice swing. There is a direct mental connection between hitting the ball and the performance.

You need to intentionally shape the way that you look at yourself in the mirror!

What if I told you that you have power to visualize an accomplishment, and through your visualization, you were able to perform just like you visualized it? You will never accomplish what you don't have a vision for. **You will never be successful in your health and fitness journey if you can't visualize yourself being successful. Your formation is the translation of what you see in the mirror!** Success doesn't fall on your lap with luck. It happens because you first visualized it, you reached for it, and you grabbed it!

Still not convinced at how powerful the mind is? Let's talk hypnosis. Hypnosis, or hypnotherapy, is the controlled suggestion of thought. Do you want to know what some of the most common reasons are for people to use hypnotherapy? The most common reason that people use hypnotherapy is to alleviate pain. The control of your thoughts can actually decrease physical pain. Another reason people seek hypnotherapy is to change behaviors such as addictions. You can change the behaviors that you act upon through the controlled suggestion of your thoughts. Another reason people use hypnotherapy is to help with physical skin conditions. It is possible to change physical conditions through the controlled suggestion of your thoughts. Your mind is responsible for pain, addictions, behaviors, and even some physical conditions. While it is complex, pain, addictions, behaviors, and even some physical conditions can be controlled through your mind.

On the topic of movies, television, and hypnosis, movies and television can produce not just suggestions but can produce what experts will call autohypnosis. Autohypnosis is a trance-like state that makes you even more susceptible to suggestion. For example, if an actor starts eating on your favorite television show, it can actually have a subliminal effect on increasing your own appetite. The media can induce autohypnosis. Because of this, eating in front of a television can lead to "mindless eating." It will have a profound impact on you if you can develop an awareness of the suggestions having a negative subliminal impact on you.

There have been multiple studies done on placebo drugs. In 2014, Novartis Consumer Health Inc funded a case study on the use of headache medicine and placebo drugs to cure headaches. It was a multi-center, double-blind, randomized, parallel-group, placebo-controlled, single-dose study. Participants at random were administered either acetaminophen at 400 mg, ibuprofen at 500 mg, or a placebo for acute treatment of headaches. A placebo drug is a fake drug with no medicinal benefit given to a controlled group during a blind study. In this study, people receiving the placebo drug don't realize that they are receiving a placebo drug and are told only that they are being administered a headache medication. In a blind study done for headaches using ibuprofen, acetaminophen, a placebo and in a time allotment of two hours, about 60 percent of individuals who were given ibuprofen reported that it relieved them of their headaches. About 52 percent of individuals who were given acetaminophen reported that it relieved them of their headaches. And about 38 percent of individuals who were given the placebo reported that it relieved them of their headaches. The individuals who received Ibuprofen were only 22 percent more likely to have relief from a headache over those who received a placebo drug. (Goldstein, 2014). While this does prove the effectiveness of a drug, it also proves the effectiveness of a belief in producing change at a physical level. There are multiple studies that have been done with placebo drugs, for a large variety of ailments, that have identified benefit from a placebo drug. How's that even possible? Instilling a thought in someone's mind that a drug is going to help them with an ailment led to a decrease in symptoms or even a cure from the ailment. How much more can you control through your mind?

The Power of Optimism

The University of Pennsylvania did a study on success prediction. In their studies, they were able to identify that there was a thinking pattern that was predictive of someone's success. That thinking pattern is optimism.

Do your thoughts usher a positive optimistic worldview, or a negative pessimistic worldview? If the mind is a battlefield, then the frontline of this battle is to create optimism and shut down pessimism. Optimism views a negative event as a temporary obstacle to be overcome and an opportunity for growth. Pessimism views a negative event as a roadblock and a setback. In the study from the University of Pennsylvania, they mentioned that there were a few behaviors attached to those who possess optimism: 1. Reaction- they were more likely to react. 2. Grit- they were more likely to endure through hardship. 3. Happiness- they were generally more excitable. And in their study, they made claim that above all other ways, there is one way to create and secure greater optimism. That way is thanksgiving, or having gratitude. The study even suggested the value of having a gratitude journal. The spirit of gratitude will change your attitude.

While it may seem farfetched, it has been proven that you will rewire your brain based on the thoughts you reflect on. **Neuroscience research has proven that your thinking patterns result in altering the physical structure and chemical balance within your brain.** As described in a neuroscience journal, "A thought can be described as the activation of a specific array of neurons. Any time a particular set of neurons is activated (sequence of thoughts), it strengthens the connections amongst these neurons. Neurons that fire together, survive together, and wire together. Because of this strengthening, the same neural pattern (thought pattern) is more likely to become active again in the future." (Siegel, 1999).

If you can learn to be grateful for the small things that you have, you'll learn to be grateful for the small achievements you create. A grateful attitude creates a self-awareness of your successes. It creates a self-awareness of what you have. What's more empowering than recognizing your achievements and successes? Thanksgiving is the simple solution to rewiring your brain and enhancing optimism. Thanksgiving will shut down a pessimistic life approach, to make way for an optimistic life approach. It steers attention away from the negative, and creates focus on the positive. The outcome is positive when the attitude is positive.

Your meditations can change your destiny. A healthy mind creates a healthy life. In fact, a pessimistic lifestyle is even associated with a greater degree of illness and a shorter life expectancy. This is due to a higher risk of health issues and the less likelihood of seeking medical help. If you want to become a new healthier version of you, it starts with a new mindset. Pessimism is an easier worldview to slip into, while being optimistic sometimes requires effort and fight. But possibly the most crucial fight is in combating your inner negativity. **Your positive mindset draws on good destiny in the same way that confidence creates a greater physical attraction.**

You are transformed by what you renew your mind with.

How does this translate? New thoughts lead to new actions. New actions lead to new habits. New habits lead to new outcomes. This is the order of change and transformation. In fact, I will refer to this order as "The 4-Step Evolution of Change." The four steps are

Thoughts, Actions, Habits, Outcomes. New thoughts lead to new actions. These "thoughts" are about yourself and your capabilities. Continued actions lead to new habits. These "actions" are the manifestation of what you believe to be possible. When new habits are formed, new outcomes are produced. These "habits" are what you do frequently and naturally. These "outcomes" are the product of a new identity. Change is a progression. This pattern of change and transformation is the sure path to successful and sustainable change. New outcomes cannot happen without new habits. New habits will never form without new actions, new actions won't begin until your thoughts change. *As you think, so you are.*

(Diagram- Evolution of Change)

Thoughts ⟶ Actions ⟶ Habits ⟶ Outcomes

The real battleground is in your head! It's time to fight the fight of thought and take captive your thoughts. How is your thought life? Is it healthy? Is it poor? Is it positive? Those thoughts are the seeds that produce change. You'll reap the seeds that you sow. If you can win in your mind, you can win in almost everything in life. It's time to discuss the evolution of change. This is what we are going to uncover together over the next two chapters.

-Chapter 5-
Turn Thoughts into Actions

"You must learn a new way to think before you can master a new way to be."
-Marianne Williamson

I can tell you with the utmost confidence where you will be in one year from now, based on how you think! Those very thoughts that you are meditating on are the very thoughts that are shaping your future and shaping your destiny. If you want to become a new healthier version of you, it starts with new thoughts. Successful thoughts lead to a successful outcome. Healthy thoughts lead to a healthy outcome. Optimistic thoughts lead to an optimistic outcome. What is your thought life like? Is it positive? Is it negative? If you want to meet your future self, look in the mirror of your current thought processes! You'll become who think you are and what you think you deserve. Let's discuss Steps 1 and 2 of "The 4 Step Evolution of Change." Step 1 being Thoughts, Step 2 being Actions.

New thoughts are the starting line to creating new outcomes! I've never met someone that completely changed their physical physique without first creating a new mind. I'm not just talking about those dramatic results, I'm talking about a change so great that there has been a shift in identity. It's the change so great that the picture of them from two years ago bears no resemblance. It's the new vocabulary, it's the new confidence, it's the new attitude, it's the new appearance. **The greatest change that can be achieved is to become unrecognizable.**

Take Control of Your Thoughts

The key element about thoughts that I'd like to bring attention to is this- Your thought life is one hundred percent controllable. While you may not have the power to control every thought that comes through your mind, every thought is a message that can either be received or declined. With every message, you can either receive it, meditate on it, then believe it, or you can immediately shut it down and delete it. You will become the thoughts that you receive and meditate on. **It's not just the thoughts that determine who you will become, it's the thoughts that you agree with.**

In the evolution of change, a change in your thought processes undeniably requires a lot of fight and discipline. It's the constant battle in and for the mind because thoughts are constant. This step requires constantly taking captive your thoughts and asking the questions: Do my thoughts bring me closer to my goals? Do they take me further from my goals? Do my thoughts build up my confidence or tear down my confidence? Do my thoughts create a high or low perspective?

On a side note, your surroundings are important in the development of your thought processes as well. There are a lot of external factors that are going to impact your thought life and many will have a subliminal impact. Your work environment will impact your thought life. Does your work environment build up your inner self or does it make you feel less than? The family and friends around you will impact your thought life. Do they promote success and believe in you, or do they make you feel like a failure? The media that you consume will impact your thought life. Does it build you up or tear you down by stirring up negativity?

The Power of Declaration

I'm assuming that since you are reading this book, you're just like me. You are hungry to grow into a greater version of yourself and eager for improvement. Because I'm hungry to grow into a greater version of myself and hungry for improvement, I guard what information and thoughts I consume. I constantly access my thought processes. If I find that my current thought processes don't align with where I envision that I'd like to be, I'll take a look in the mirror and speak declarations over myself. As I mentioned in my bio, my life was forever changed when Cynthia Corder handed me an "I am" declaration sheet and told me to declare these "I am's" over my life every single day. There was nothing more pivotal in my recovery process as a teenager than the creation of new thoughts. I began to see myself differently. It was central in my transformation journey from being a destructive teenager to becoming an influential motivational speaker who taught others how to become free from addiction in the span of just a few years. I'm going to give you this practical tactic, and it's a tactic that I still use to this day. Create positive self-declarations. I'm going to be vulnerable with you. I actually have a list of "I can, I will, I am" declarations that I frequently declare over myself. Here's an example of what my declaration list that I speak over myself might look like based on an assessment of my thought processes. There is undeniably power in what you declare over yourself as it generates a lot of power over your thought processes. I'll even look at myself in the mirror and repeat these declarations until I start to see myself differently.

If I find myself doubting my ability to be successful.... "I can be successful, I will be successful, I am successful"

If I find myself thinking lazy thoughts and not wanting to workout.... "I can conquer my workouts this week, I will conquer my workouts this week, I am a conqueror"

If I find myself allowing fear to hold me back from pursuing my dreams... "I can be courageous toward accomplishing my dreams, I will be courageous toward accomplishing my dreams, I am courageous"

If I find myself not wanting to eat healthy... "I can eat healthy, I will eat healthy, I am healthy"

If I find myself procrastinating... "I can be disciplined in my work tasks this week, I will be disciplined in my work tasks this week, I am disciplined"

If I find myself thinking about temptations from previous addictions.... "I can be free from addictions, I will be free from addictions, I am free"

If I find myself allowing too many distractions... "I can be focused on my goals, I will be focused on my goals, I am focused"

"Whatever we plant in our subconscious mind and nourish with repetition and emotion will one day become a reality." -Earl Nightingale

In 1949, neuropsychologist Donald Hebb described how pathways in the brain are formed and reinforced. The brain is wired through repetition. The more the brain does a certain task, the stronger that neural network becomes, making the process more efficient each successive time. This is why the practice of gratitude is so effective. The repetition of gratitude changes neural patterns.

On November 25, 1835, a child was born who would one day become the richest man in the world. His name was Andrew Carnegie. In Andrew's teenage years, a mentor, recognizing Andrew's ambitions to be successful, gave Andrew a very profound piece of advice. He told Andrew that if he wants to become rich, everyday he needs to look at himself in the mirror and declare over himself "I will be the richest man in the world." It was documented that he made claim of how unrealistic it seemed at first when he was making those declarations. Then one day, a switch happened. His belief started to transform, and he started to recognize that it was realistic to become the richest man in the world. It has been documented that the more he began to declare this message over himself, the more he began to believe it. Through owning the steel industry at the peak of the Industrial Revolution, he one day became the richest man in the world. Experts today estimate that his net worth in today's economy would be between $300-$400 billion dollars, making him one of the richest men to ever live.

What if I told you that you can have greater success in life simply by creating optimistic and positive declarations? While the declarations may not seem to yield much power, the most profound impact that these declarations produce is a new belief. Andrew Carnegie didn't magically become successful simply from telling himself that he would be. It was out of his newly created belief system that it became a possibility. And because of his strong belief system it became a reality. **Your capacity for success is one hundred percent dictated by your belief. You will only be able to achieve what your mind first believes.** If you believe that you can't do something, you have almost a zero percent chance of that achievement. If you believe that you can do something, you've entered into the realm of possibility. Nothing is impossible if there is first a belief.

Create New Belief

If your belief system says "I am a loser," it'll be hard to win. If your belief system says "I am a winner," it'll be hard to lose. From the moment that you wake up, are your thoughts "I'm going to conquer my day" or "I'm just going to get through my day"? It will make a huge difference on how you act and perform. While it may seem cliche to create a declaration sheet, when you declare and meditate on such thoughts, the mind is rewired and new beliefs are created.

"It's the repetition of affirmations that lead to belief. And once that belief becomes a deep conviction, things begin to happen." -Muhammad Ali.

The goal with these new thoughts is to create a new belief system. The repetition of thoughts become belief. And most importantly, the belief will provoke new actions. This is the next step in the evolution of change. New thoughts lead to new actions. You'll act on what you believe to be possible, and you won't even attempt something that you don't believe to be possible.

(Diagram- Thoughts/Beliefs/Actions)

Thoughts ➡➡➡ Belief ➡➡➡ Actions

"Behind every system of actions is a system of beliefs."
- James Clear

How does this relate to your health and fitness goals? If there is not a true belief that you have the capability to reach your goal of dropping 30 pounds of body fat, there will be no possibility. If you don't believe that you can put on 20 pounds of muscle, there will be no possibility. If you don't believe that you can change your lifestyle, a change in lifestyle is not a possibility.

The repetition of your thoughts is about the strengthening of a new belief system. The stronger the belief system, the more likely you are to respond and act on that belief system. Actions are nothing less than the physical manifestation of the belief system! There will only be progress in your actions if there is first progress in your beliefs. On the flip side, there will never be progress in your actions, without progress in your beliefs.

Motivation for You: Believe in Yourself

Henry Ford once said, "The man who thinks he can and the man who thinks he can't are both right."

Stop thinking about every reason why you can't accomplish something great, and start meditating on why you can accomplish something great. If you tell yourself that you can't, you have a zero percent chance of success. If you tell yourself that you can, you've entered into the realm of possibility. Stop thinking about how painful the tough times are, and start thinking about how tough times are making you stronger. Same thing in your workouts. Stop thinking about how painful each rep is, and start thinking about how the pain is making you stronger. It's so easy to think negatively, but if you can adjust your mindset and view all those negative things as a positive, you'll rewire your brain. That same thought pattern is more likely to become active in the future. If you meditate on "I can," "I can" will become the natural firing thought when faced with the question of "can I?" If you meditate on "I will," "I will" will become the natural firing thought when faced with the question of "will I?" If you meditate on "I am," "I am" will become the natural firing thought when faced with the question of "am I?" If you can take control of your mind, you can take control of your life.

The front line of the war is in your head, so fight the fight of thought. **If something has the ability to be thought provoking, that would suggest that you have the ability to provoke thought.** Start provoking thoughts. If you want to transform your life, think intentionally. Most people don't lead their life, they accept their life. That's a fixed mindset. Don't accept your thoughts. Lead your thoughts. Leading your thought life gives your brain a positive and healthy promotion. That's a growth mindset.

Your thoughts are nothing less than the ceiling of your capabilities. You can't expect to become a new man and still think like the old man. Don't expect a different outcome by doing the same things you've always done. Don't expect a different outcome by thinking the same things you've always thought. That's the definition of insanity! If you are embracing the "thoughts of your past," you can't expect to take a hold of a different future. In reference to these thoughts, I'm talking about what you think you can accomplish, what you think you will accomplish, and who you think you are. You won't even swing the bat if you don't think you can hit the ball. **Optimism generates the idea of "I can." Determination generates the idea of "I will." Confidence generates the idea of "I am."**

A strong belief system will shift, "I can, I will, I am" into "I must." One of the strongest powers that you can possess is the belief system of "I must." You won't automatically act differently from new beliefs as every aspect of the process does require effort. But when the belief becomes "I must," actions become a necessity. Imagine how profound of an impact it will make on your success rate when new actions become a necessity. Creating new actions will become just as important as breathing is to you. "I must do this to survive!"

Don't ever let someone tell you what you can and cannot achieve. Success is your decision. Nobody else's. You have every resource and tool you need to be successful. The biggest tool is a belief system. It doesn't matter what a friend said about you. It doesn't matter what your boss said about you. It doesn't even matter what a family member said about you. The only thing that matters is what you say about you. Who cares who they say you are. You are who YOU say you are. "I am who I say I am. I am!...." You've got to do whatever it takes to create those new beliefs. It starts with guarding your mind! Take a look in the mirror everyday and remind yourself of who you really are! The one person who will determine your success is the person that looks back at you in the mirror every morning when you wake up. Don't wait for everyone else to start believing in you. Nobody is going to fully believe in you, until you fully believe in yourself. Nothing is impossible for he/she who believes! See it, think it, believe it, go achieve it, and then repeat it!

-Chapter 6-
Create a Great Outcome

"The outcome of the highest achievement is an identity change."
-Trey Patterson

Continued actions lead to new habits. In this chapter, I'm going to discuss Steps 3 and 4 of the 4-Step Evolution of Change. Step 3 being Habits and Step 4 being Outcomes.

Here are my two favorite definitions of a habit according to the Miriam Webster dictionary. "1. A settled tendency or a usual manner of behavior. 2. A behavior pattern acquired by frequent repetition of physiological exposure that shows itself in regularity or increased facility of performance." It's an action that has become a regular practice. The first thing that I'd like to point out is that a habit can be formed by frequent repetition. You're probably recognizing a trend here. Repetition. Repetition of thoughts, repetition of actions, leads to the natural firing repetition of actions (habit). It's as simple as brushing your teeth right before bed. It becomes the natural firing action when it's your last trip to the bathroom before heading to bed. Or it's the natural firing actions that take place in the shower. I wash my hair, then put conditioner in my hair, then wash my body, then rinse out my conditioner, then wash my face, then turn the cold water on for one minute, then dry off. There's no thought to my actions when in the shower; they are just natural firing actions because of formed habits.

Create Strong Habits

There are three factors that make a habit strong. 1. Frequency. How often do you perform the habit? 2. Duration of the habit. How long have you been engaging in the habit? A few weeks, several months, many years? 3. The pleasure you receive from the habit. Is the habit enjoyable? The more you enjoy it the stronger the desire to continue the habit. **The more that you enjoy something, the more you do something, and the longer the duration of time that you've been doing it, the harder it is to break the habit and change your actions.**

The biggest mistake I see with fitness New Years resolutioners is they go from 0 to 100 mph in a short duration of time. Let's use the New Years resolutioner as the illustration. They have high frequency. Meaning they start going to the gym maybe 3-4 days a week. Naturally, they have low duration. They just started going to the gym a few weeks prior on January 1st. And, they have little to no pleasure in their exercise and diet regiment. This is a recipe for disaster. Ninety percent of these New Years resolutioners won't have much success. They rely on self-motivation to pull them through to success. While motivation is powerful, it's also very fickle, and it will come and go. There will be days where you are not motivated and for some, entire seasons where you will lack any motivation. The goal is to successfully form a habit and be prepared for your season of low motivation!

The number one ingredient to creating a strong habit of exercise is enjoying or finding pleasure in the form of exercise of participation. Maybe the reason you're stuck in a plateau is because you've lost your enjoyment. You may lose a good habit by losing your enjoyment. Fitness and exercise are physical, and you must find what you physically enjoy. All this talk of trying new forms of exercise or foods is a part of the action step of the Evolution of Change, but it is vital in understanding how to create new habits. Now for some, arguably a large percentage of us, the pleasure may not necessarily come from the feelings of the exercise itself, but the pleasure comes from the benefits of the exercise regimen. Through time, you'll gain pleasure through seeing results. You'll get pleasure in knowing you're getting stronger. You'll get pleasure in knowing you've lost several inches in your waist. Your pleasures and reasons for enjoyment might change, but you must always find your reasons to enjoy what you are doing.

Great habits lead to great outcomes. When I meditate on habits, the first thing that I think of is having good financial habits. I'm going to steer our attention toward habits in a financial realm then come full circle. I'm going to use a couple of the wealthiest men in the world as an illustration to prove my point. Elon Musk lives in a tiny home. He said, "This house is comfortable and it's all I need." Jeff Bezos, when he became a billionaire was still driving a Honda Civic. He said, "The car is a good and reliable car." At the start of 2023, Elon Musk and Jeff Bezos were the two richest men in the world. The richest men/women in the world got to where they are because of good habits. Their success wasn't simply through making a lot of money in their business, but in creating good financial habits. I'm about to come full circle with this. Don't expect a great outcome if you sell yourself for what's temporary and doesn't add value. Only sell yourself on that which brings value. Bad habits lead to bad outcomes. If you have a habit of eating junk food, don't expect to have a good outcome. If you develop a habit of meal prepping and exercise, you are bound to have a good outcome.

The harsh reality is that it's easier to slip into unhealthy habits than it is to develop healthy habits. Like eating fast food, unhealthy habits are almost always cheap and easy. Starting a healthy habit is hard, but the more you practice it, the easier it becomes. **Practice doesn't make perfect, practice makes permanent.** Be intentional and disciplined in your practices.

It takes time to form new habits. Just how long? Let's take it back to the old school. In 1960, a cosmetic surgeon named Dr. Maxwell Maltz wrote a self-help book called "Psycho Cybernetics, A New Way to Get More Living Out of Life." Within his book, he talks about habits, how habits are formed, and how he developed the 21/90 formula. He suggested that it takes 21 days to form a new habit, and it takes 90 days to break an old habit. The good news is that it doesn't take long to form a habit. However, it does take longer to break a habit. The reason I'm sharing this is because it's important to understand that a change in habits takes time. It requires commitment.

Habits never form overnight. Assuming that a new belief system has compelled new actions and you now have a goal of maintaining these new actions, I'm going to give you a practical tool to help form a new habit. The most powerful tool that you can use to form a new habit is in the formation of routines. Routines are created. You can make the decision to start a new routine tomorrow, but you can't start a new habit tomorrow. Habits are the natural firing reaction.

Form a Routine

Let's discuss the subconscious effect of forming a habit through creating a routine using an alarm clock as an illustration. Let's say that you get into the routine of setting your alarm to 6 a.m. every morning, and you stay consistent. For the first few weeks, your alarm clock will wake you up. Over time your body begins to change and your biological clock will begin to shift. Your body will eventually create a natural response to waking up around the scheduled time and will habitually wake up around 6 a.m. What started as a routine, formed a habit. Flip it around, this is even how unhealthy habits are formed. Let's take drug addiction for an example. If everyday at 7 p.m. you pop a pill to get high, after a month straight of that routine–more than 21 days as a measurement of duration– it then becomes a habit. If you stop cold turkey after 21 days of continuous use, the next day your body will crave it around 7 p.m. A pleasurable habit, a frequent habit, and a high duration habit of several months to years can lead to full blown addiction. A key element to breaking that addiction is forming new thoughts and new routines.

(Diagram: Actions/Routines/Habits)

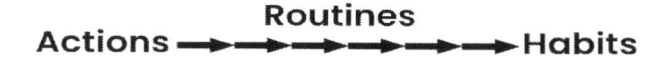

Actions ⟶⟶⟶ Routines ⟶⟶ Habits

Sometimes creating new routines won't excite you. That's the nature of the beast. But the goal is for the routine to produce a habit. Let's take eating junk food at lunchtime for example. Let's say you get an hour break, and you get into the routine of grabbing lunch at a junk food chain. That routine will then become a habit of eating junk food for lunch, and when noon strikes, your body will begin to crave junk food. At 9 p.m. you turn on the television to watch your favorite show. While watching your favorite show, you get into the routine of eating unhealthy snacks. That routine will eventually lead to a habit, and every time that you turn on that favorite show at 9 p.m., your body will habitually start to crave that unhealthy snack. It's not the hunger that stimulates the cravings for junk food, it's the routine that formed the habit of eating junk food. That's the power of habit. Your habits produce the cravings.

Now, staying consistent in a routine works in another way. Routines help keep your habits consistent. If you stop setting your alarm clock for 6 a.m., your body may shift away from waking itself up around 6 a.m. If you need to get up at 6 a.m., you will still set an alarm clock as that will allow you to wake up precisely when you need to.

Breaking a Habit

On the topic of forming a habit, I think it's equally important to discuss how to break a habit. Let's discuss breaking a habit in terms of breaking an addiction. An addiction is more complex than a habit, as with any addiction there is a psychological dependency to the habit. But I do believe that the concepts of breaking an addiction can translate to breaking a habit. If these concepts can work for an addiction, they can surely work for a habit.

If one of the factors in making a habit strong is the enjoyment or pleasure that comes from the habit, then I believe the starting line for ending a habit/addiction is through "unpleasant experience" or in psychological terms creating negative reinforcement. If a habit can be linked to an unpleasant or negative experience, there will be a greater desire to eliminate that habit. Simply put, if you don't desire change, you probably won't change. In an addiction realm, in most cases, the individual will need to have an unpleasant experience, or a series of unpleasant experiences, that are connected to their habit in order to desire change. A counselor may suggest to a family member or friend that in order for their loved one to break their addiction, they must have a "rock bottom" experience that produces the desire to change. I believe the number one reason that people seek to break a habit or addiction is because they no longer enjoy it.

While it may sound cliché, identify your reasons to dislike your unhealthy habits.

Breaking addiction can be very complex and challenging. In some cases of severe addiction, there is not just a psychological dependency but there is also a physiological dependency. One thing that is extremely important to note, whether it comes to breaking a severe addiction or a simple habit, is the impact of triggers. A trigger is any stimulus that connects an individual to a habit or addiction and can elicit a response or relapse. **Triggers are one hundred percent encoded in your environment.** A familiar environment will trigger familiar habits. While the friends around you can be a trigger, your environment stretches far beyond people. The music you listen to, the video games you play, the television and movies that you watch can be a trigger as well and can offer strong suggestions. Listening to the same music that you listened to ten years ago can keep pulling you back into your past behaviors. This is done because feelings, emotions, and memories are connected to music.

One of the most powerful things that you can do in the creation of a new environment is developing an awareness of what triggers you. Let's simplify this. Let's say that you are trying to end the habit of eating fast food. Something must trigger the desire to eat fast food. Sure, hunger is going to trigger it. Side note, you can prevent that trigger by making the decision to eat something healthy if you know you are about to start getting hungry. Learn to recognize your triggers and cut off the source and availability. Maybe it's watching TV during prime time. Avoid watching that prime time show during prime time. Those fast food commercials strategically come on during prime time because they know it's dinner time and you may be hungry. It's successful marketing. Maybe it's driving a certain route home where you pass the routine fast food joint. Avoid the route of passing that routine fast food restaurant, because that trigger may elicit a response.

In cases of severe addiction, a clean house is of extreme importance in the success rate of breaking an addiction. My victory over drug addiction in my teenage years was produced because of multiple reasons. Apart from having a rock-bottom experience in a jail cell and going through the 12 Steps of AA, I had a complete change in environment by spending eight months in a military school instead of my prior school. And I made new friends and moved into a new house. I not only had the desire to change, but I had a complete change in my environment. And, during this time I gave my life to Christ and created a relationship with God which promoted my lifestyle and environment changes. I practiced renewing my mind to form a new identity. I stopped listening to the old music that I previously listened to, I stopped playing the old video games that I previously played, and stopped watching the same movies and television shows that I watched prior. I even stopped dating for a few years as the emotions from dating were triggers for me. My triggers had been eliminated.

If you seriously desire change, you've got to get serious about changing your environment!

If your kitchen looks just like it did before you went on the quest to form new healthy eating habits, it will be a trigger. So many of us need to do routine kitchen sweeps to get rid of unhealthy foods. Familiar environments produce memories and triggers. The wrong environment creates an uphill battle, while the elimination of triggers is about creating a downhill battle. It's about creating systems that make success easy. You can make the battle so much more challenging by being in the wrong environment. It's time to radically change your environment!

Your Greatest Outcome

Now, within the 4-Step Evolution of Change, Step 3 is new habits and Step 4 is new outcomes. Step 4, being new outcomes, seems pretty self-explanatory right? New outcomes come from new habits. It means new accomplishments. It means new results. It means new successes. But, it also means something deeper. New outcomes are the formation of a new identity. **The outcome of the highest achievement is an identity change.** The ultimate end goal is to create a new identity. What's the difference in "healthy eating" and a "healthy eater"? Healthy eating is a habit; healthy eater is an identity.

(Diagram: Habits/Identity/Outcomes)

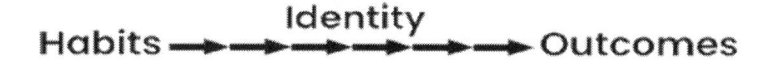

Habits → → Identity → → → Outcomes

Research has proven that when your identity becomes attached to your habit, you'll be more likely to continue in that habit. In fact, there is a term used to describe behavior and habit prediction, called Identity Behavior Theory (IBT). In simplicity, if you think you're a criminal, you'll act like a criminal. If you tell a kid everyday that they are bad, they are more likely to act out behaviors that reflect their shaped identities.

Don't seek to get into the routine of cycling, seek to become a cyclist. Don't seek to start running, seek to become a runner. Don't seek to start reading, seek to become a reader. Do you see the difference? Identity! Cycling is the habit; cyclist is the outcome. Running is the habit; runner is the outcome. Reading is the habit; reader is the outcome. Don't just seek to form a new habit, seek to form a new identity. Don't just practice it, become it! **When you become it, you are more likely to create a sustainable transformation.**

The more you practice habits, the more it changes your identity. Just like how the duration of an action makes a habit strong, the duration of the habit makes the identity strong. The longer that you engage in your habit, the more it becomes attached to your identity and the more it will distinguish you. Transformation is about constantly stepping into a new identity. The goal is to develop a new identity, then develop a greater identity, then an even greater identity.

This leads me to my next point, developing a new identity is a long process. For some, it's shorter. For some, it takes longer. If you already eat fairly clean meals, it may take you less time to develop an identity of clean eater than someone who primarily eats fast food. It could take the latter several years to develop an identity of clean eater as they'll have a much longer process. For someone who was raised in extreme poverty, it will take them longer to develop an identity of rich as opposed to someone who was raised in the middle class. For some, the evolution of change is a long process. The only requirement for success in the change in identity is that you don't quit on the process!

I'm no longer a recovering drug addict! I'm a new creation and a new man with changed desires. I have a new identity! **The 4-Step Evolution of Change summarized in two words is "identity process."** It's the evolution of the new identity.

You'll think new thoughts and see new things. You'll act on what you see and believe. You'll practice what you see and believe until it becomes habit. Then through habit reoccurrence, you become! That is how the greatest transformations are produced! If you want to dramatically change your life, you need to develop a new identity. This is the heartbeat of a new outcome and the greatest way to create sustainable change.

If you want to grow into the best version of your future self, it requires intention in your actions today. But what good are those actions if you haven't changed who you are? More than likely you'll eventually revert back to who you think you are and what you think you deserve. If you can destroy old habits and form new habits, you will create new outcomes! If you can continue in those habits, you'll eventually form a new identity. The greatest outcome achieved is the changing of an identity. By definition, transformation is the constant change in identity. Just like at a molecular level, when a transformation of a cell take place, it will never revert back to its previous structure. It's the constant game of destroying the old to make room for the new. And it's constantly becoming a greater you! Keep it constant, and constantly you will change and transform!

-Chapter 7-
Enjoy The Process

"The reality is, everyone likes exercise and for those who say they don't, they just haven't been on the quest of discovery."
-Trey Patterson

Diet culture has given us the illusion that transformation is a short and quick process. "Here's my 30-day before and after transformation." This short-term perception of transformation can lead to unhealthy habits and unhealthy behaviors. Transformation is a process and the process is the most important part of the journey. It's the place where we discover what we enjoy. It's the place where we discover who we are. It's the place where we create our environment. The process is where habits are formed and new disciplines are created. The process is our development. And finally, the process is the journey to a new outcome!

The 4-Step Evolution of Change are the stages in which transformation happens. **The process is the systems that you create to make transformation happen.**

First, let's bring the definition of process back to our attention. According to Oxford Languages, process is defined as "a series of actions or steps taken in order to achieve a particular end."

When discussing the process, I'm talking about the actions and steps taken to become successful in your health and fitness transformation journey. Over the next four chapters, I'm going to talk about the important elements within the process of transformation that you can control. The outcome is the product of what you control through the process. The process is about seeking out what you enjoy and what brings you pleasure. The process is about creating the right environment. The process is about developing discipline. And in all complexity, the process is ongoing and ever changing.

There are two words that create magic within the process- Finding Enjoyment!

Before I continue within the subsection on the process, I would like to mention that in this chapter and Chapter 9, I will be speaking to a slightly different audience. This is because everyone is in a different place within the process of change and transformation. Everyone is in a different point in their journey. In this chapter, I'm going to speak directly to the individual that struggles finding the motivation to even get started in their regimen and/or is new to their regimen. And in Chapter 9, I'm going to speak to the individual that may be further in the process and/or struggles to stay committed long-term.

My Personal Mistakes

I'm going to begin by talking about an unhealthy element in my personal bodybuilding journey. When I was 25 years old, I started competing in men's physique bodybuilding competitions. I would compete in four competitions over the next four years of my life. As a competitive bodybuilder, I had a very strict exercise and dieting routine while on prep. My average competition prep duration was about 12 weeks. During the first four to six weeks of a prep, I would go through a bulk phase where I would consume a large number of calories. For me it was between 5,000-6,000 calories per day with the goal of putting on as much size as possible, body fat and muscle. I could successfully gain between 15-20 pounds within the first six weeks. Then, four to six weeks before my show, I would begin a cut phase with the goal of dropping body fat while preserving muscle. I could successfully drop about 8-10 pounds of mostly body fat within my last six weeks. During this time, I would count my macros to an exact measurement and have to eat very specific meals and portions. Truthfully, I absolutely hated those last four to six weeks. Eating extremely healthy, portion-controlled meals for a short duration put a really bad taste in my mouth toward healthy eating. When the show was over, I would rebound and I would be back to eating junk food. And when I use the term "eating junk food," I'm referring to me giving my appetite all power over my eating decisions and eating whatever I wanted. Eating foods that I hated for four weeks without any "cheat meals" made that pizza after my competition taste much better. Because of this fitness journey approach, this rebound led to me enjoying junk food even more. Within a month, I would easily put back on ten pounds of body fat. I can honestly say that during this time of doing competitions, I developed a very unhealthy relationship with food.

  In regards to my workout regimen, I would go from working out three times per week in the off-season of competition to working out ten times per week during prep season. Yes, that means multiple two times per day workouts a week. I created an extreme change knowing that it wasn't something I was going to sustain long-term yet would yield dramatic results. Mind you, prior to my competition days, I would comfortably workout roughly five times per week as it was something that I really enjoyed. I can honestly say that making these extreme changes in my workout regimen actually led to me developing an unhealthy relationship with exercise as well. From working out ten times per week, I lost my enjoyment as it became something I had to do, rather than wanted to do. After a competition, I dreaded going to the gym, and it was a fight for me to still workout three times per week. You can imagine that going from eating a very strict diet and working out ten times per week, to eating junk food and working out three times per week led to a dramatic body composition change.

There is something vital that I would like to point out here. **I believe the reason that a lot of people struggle with their fitness goals is because their fitness journey is very similar to my competition prep journey. You're trying to create a dream physique in 12 weeks!** Stop trying to force new actions especially if you don't enjoy these new actions. Possibly the most important element of being successful in your health and fitness journey is finding enjoyment in the process.

I'm not bashing the sport of bodybuilding as I did enjoy how it challenged me mentally and how it pushed me into strict discipline. And I'm not bashing the individual who is trying to get dramatic results in a short time span to get ready for a vacation, wedding, or competition. That's not the audience that this message is for. I'm speaking to the individual who is in the pursuit of sustainable change.

For me, there was a very unhealthy element to my competition prep journey. It made me develop very unhealthy patterns. Those four years of competing consisted of extreme highs of me standing on stage feeling great about my physique to extreme lows where I would look at myself in the mirror and be disgusted by what I saw. I did develop body dysmorphia. I felt like I was always trying to get back to where I used to be. When I eventually got tired of looking the way that I was looking, I would then sign up for another competition to start my "12-week transformation" with the goal of looking as good or even better than in my previous competition. I developed an unhealthy perception of myself, and I would undergo extreme changes and do whatever it took to have the best physique. These extreme patterns within my competition journey led to a very unhealthy version of me. I was the one who made this decision to create these patterns, initially thinking it would make me "better." Little did I know, it wasn't setting me up to become "better" long-term. I thought that setting a 12-week goal to stand up on a stage in a men's physique competition would force me to eat cleaner, workout more, and essentially become healthier. What I was actually doing was creating short-term solutions while not effectively fixing the root of the problem. **The root of the problem was solely in an obsessive fixation on the outcome, rather than learning and implementing personal development through the process.** What I really needed was to create a new sustainable lifestyle.

  The reason that I'm sharing about my four years of competition prep journey and my personal struggles is because I think that a majority of people can relate to my experience in their health and fitness journey, in some form or fashion. Some of us can relate to beating ourselves down because of an unhappiness with our appearance. Some of us can even relate to the positive feeling of receiving validation from someone else. And many of us can relate to that roller coaster of constantly trying to get back to where we were. Twelve weeks before that vacation we jump on the fad diet and start exercising once again. It feels like a constant game of getting back to that high of having that great physique, and it is because we've created a series of unhealthy patterns that have led to the roller coaster effect. If we are not careful, we can condition ourselves to have a bad relationship with exercise and food.

I have a personal training client named Desiree. She is a client that inspires me as she not only has very strong discipline, but she enjoys healthy eating and exercising five times or more per week. The most important factor in her fitness journey success is she truthfully enjoys a healthy lifestyle. She doesn't have to force herself to eat clean or exercise. At 41 years old, she stood on a stage and competed in an NPC bikini competition. Not only did she place in two divisions, but she smoked girls half her age. Her physique didn't develop through 12 weeks of hard training. It came through several years of creating a healthy lifestyle and actually finding enjoyment in this healthy lifestyle. She has learned the art of falling in love with the process. **Falling in love with the process makes the arrival of the destination much easier.**

Try Something New

"But Trey, I hate exercise!" I would say that close to 25 percent of my onboarding personal training clients admit this. Come to find out, they just haven't had previous pleasurable experiences with strength training or cardio. But, one hundred percent of the time, they eventually come to recognize that they do like at least a few forms of exercise. Exercise extends beyond strength training and cardio and includes all physical activity. The reality is, everyone likes exercise and for those who say they don't, they just haven't been on the quest of discovery.

Your newly established thoughts and confidence in becoming successful will compel you to step out and try new things. People dread a diet because that means they must eat what they don't want to eat. At a psychological level, who wants to be on a diet? Try different kinds of healthy foods and you'll find something healthy that you really enjoy. Sometimes it takes trying a lot of different healthy snacks to replace those unhealthy snacks that you enjoy. Creating a new healthy menu that you enjoy is not an overnight process.

People dread an exercise regimen because they haven't found what they enjoy. If you are trying to force an exercise regimen that you don't enjoy, you'll easily get burnt out. Once a burnout occurs, re-ignition is extremely difficult. Your enjoyment is the gasoline to the fire! Give that kickboxing class a shot. Maybe you'll love strength training. If you love to dance, why aren't you taking that dance class? Try hiring a personal trainer! You'll never fully know what you like and dislike until you try it. If at first you don't succeed, dust yourself off and try something new. If you don't enjoy it, it's going to be hard to stick with it, and it will be hard to reach the destination. **While there may be some forms of exercise that are more beneficial toward specific fitness goals, it's better to find that which you enjoy, than to start something that you won't continue due to the lack of enjoyment.**

Maybe you did find an exercise regimen that you enjoyed but you are bored of it. If you are bored, I can almost guarantee you that it's because you haven't tried something new in awhile. We are always watching something new on TV, why? It's our human nature to desire something new and fresh. It's even part of the reason why sports are seasonal. You'd lose interest if it was year-round. In the same manner that you get bored watching a TV show, you'll change the channel to watch something else. Maybe you need to pick up the remote and tune into a new fitness channel. Don't get bored or burnt out from doing the same thing repetitively. Diversify your exercise experience to make sure it's always exciting for you.

Some of my most successful clients, and in terms of success, I'm referring to the clients that have created a sustainable regimen, have a very diverse exercise regimen. They'll spend a few months doing one form of exercise that they enjoy, then switch it up the following season. Some will have a gym membership for a few months at a boutique cycling gym, then will have a gym membership taking a high intensity interval training class for a few months, then have a gym membership taking a boxing class for a few months, then they circuit. All of my sports-loving clients know exactly what I'm talking about when I say this. There is a fresh excitement when the season changes and it's time for the next sport season to start, whether it's football, basketball, soccer, hockey, baseball, etc. You can create that excitement by having an exercise regimen circuit. "It's springtime, which means its cycling season!"

If you struggle to find the enjoyment in your regimen, maybe look at what time of the day you are exercising. Maybe you dislike it because you have to go after a long day at work. Try working out early in the morning. I've had many people switch from evening workouts to early morning workouts and they will report it being challenging to adjust at first, but they feel substantially better throughout the day. If you are working out early in the morning, try working out in the afternoon after you've had a couple meals. I've had many report having much more energy after working out later in the day. Everybody has a sweet spot where they feel their best and get their most effective workout. Maybe you just haven't found your sweet spot. I've had many clients that switched workout times and their energy, attitude, and even their demeanor was completely different.

If you can teach yourself to fall in love with the process, getting to your desired outcome won't be a challenge. If you can't teach yourself to fall in love with the process, you'll never be fully content with the outcome. This is what we must realize- Your growth comes from the process. Your development comes from the process. Knowledge comes from the process. Your transformation is found within the process. So don't be outcome-focused, be process-focused!

I hear a lot of weight loss clients say, "Well it's time for me to start losing weight again, it's time for me to go back on a diet and exercise regimen." That attitude about the process is something you cannot sustain and you are setting yourself up for failure. By saying "I'm going back 'on' a diet and exercise regimen," you are actually admitting to yourself that you eventually plan on going back "off" your diet and exercise regimen. Instead of going on and off a diet and exercise regimen, discover what works for you and what you enjoy. It's easy to create a lifestyle around what you enjoy and it's only when it becomes your lifestyle that it becomes sustainable. The reality is, if you want the greatest transformation, if you want the greatest growth, if you want the greatest level of success, you must change your lifestyle.

You can't expect a different outcome by doing the same things you've always done. That's insanity! Transformation starts with getting excited about what you are doing. Of course, there will be challenges in the process. Sometimes the journey can feel like a roller coaster. There will be times where you see success, and there will be times where you feel like you are failing. Don't quit on the process. The journey is the great discovery. It's where you discover who you are, what you like, and what works for you. If the journey isn't challenging, the destination won't be a reward! Embrace the process and eventually you'll receive your reward!

-Chapter 8-
Reclaim Your Environment

"Strategically choose your circle of friends because your proximity will determine your prosperity!"
-Trey Patterson

Who are you doing life with?

Every single one of us has our circle of friends. Let me take a moment and talk to you about your circle, because that circle will have a huge impact on your success. Your circle consists of the people that you do life with. They are the ones you intentionally spend time with. They are the ones that you call close friends. They are the ones whose feedback and opinions you value the most. So, who are you doing life with? Take time to really think about it. You won't go much further in life than the people you are surrounded by. If you have naysayers or people who are negative in your circle… CUT THEM OUT! A bad tree doesn't produce good fruit. Stop trying to eat the fruit of someone who isn't feeding you with the good.

Imagine being a boxer, and after a single round of defeat, you go back to your corner and have someone in your corner tell you, "Man, you lost that round, you are going to lose this fight." In the heat of the moment, a boxer who has taken hit after hit, goes back to his corner to have someone speak negativity over him while he is in his most vulnerable state. It will require a lot of will power for him to shake off the negativity and stay fully engaged and confident in his fight. Do you want to know which individuals have the most impact over you when you are in your most vulnerable state? It's your circle! The ones in your close corner. You may not realize it until you start taking inventory of your friends, but you probably have some of these negative people in your circle. When you feel down and discouraged, nobody is going to bring you down further than someone from your circle giving you the "you can't do it" vibe.

"I'm just a realist!" said every pessimist.

It's hard to stand on an upper ledge and pull someone up to you. Positivity can be overpowered by negativity. It is easy to stand on a lower ledge and pull someone down to you. If you have people in your large circle of friends that build you up and believe in you, they belong in your circle. These people are the gasoline to your fires. **Strategically choose your circle of friends because your proximity will determine your prosperity!** Your environment will determine your opportunity! If you hang out with nine successful people, there is no doubt that you will be the tenth. Do you know how much more knowledge you'll collect from hanging out with nine successful people than from hanging out with nine unsuccessful people? And of course I'm talking about success in your fitness journey. Start hanging out with nine other people who are successful in their fitness journey and see where it takes you. Put yourself in an environment where you are challenged to be the best. **You don't become a Serena Williams without a Venus in your life! You'll grow to the level of those around you.**

If you can be disciplined in who you hang out with, you can exponentially increase your likelihood of success, in any area of your life. When you cut out the bad to make room for the good in your life, you are setting the foundation for your transformation. Cultivating your environment is one of the most important pieces of the process.

The Environment of Growth

Does a crop farmer grow crops?

The correct answer is no. A crop farmer doesn't grow crops. They create an environment where crops can grow. Develop that mindset about your success. You must create an environment for success. You must remove the weeds that will choke growth. A farmer would never plant seeds in a field full of thorns and expect growth. You must have the right environment to cultivate that growth. Those people in your circle are your environment.

The second thing that I'd like to point out is, you must have the right climate to nourish growth. The attitude around you is your climate. Negativity is like a desert. With the absence of nourishment, almost nothing can grow. Positivity is like the rainforest where everything can grow. Unlike a crop farmer, luckily for you, you can control your environment and climate. You must have the right team to flourish in your growth, and a team that will grow with you. Always take inventory of your friends, and recognize those within your circle that don't promote growth.

Sometimes it's not even about being around other successful people, but it's about being around the right energy. It's not just negativity versus positivity. It's negative energy versus positive energy.

It's a powerful attribute if you can learn how to read the right energy in people. Does their presence promote your growth so that you walk away from them feeling stronger and empowered? Sometimes two successful people can be the same side of the magnet that doesn't carry the right attraction and will end up pushing each other further from success.

If you don't remove those individuals, those individuals will remove you from your goals. The reality is, if you are running hard toward success, there are people you will have to leave behind. Stop slowing down for others so that they can catch up, you've got a time goal in your race to hit. Every runner will understand this, especially those who do road races. Find the runners and stick with them in your race. Find that pacer that's going to challenge you and keep up. Don't slow down or stop for the walkers. You've got a finish line of success to get to.

As a side note, when it comes to pursuing your health and fitness goals, I would highly recommend having an accountability partner or even an accountability group. Through years of group and personal training, I've seen hundreds of accountability partners. Two is always better than one. **Having an accountability partner is the glue that keeps two people committed to their goals.** Submerse yourself in health and fitness culture by joining an accountability group. Join a Facebook group. Join a community at a gym. Be active on that health and fitness forum. If you want to be successful, surround yourself with other people with the same goals.

If you put a baby shark in a small 20-30 gallon tank, it will only grow about 8-12 inches. That same shark placed in the ocean can easily grow to eight feet. That's about 10 times the length and at least 40-50 times the weight. For some of us, the reason we are not reaching our full capabilities is because we are not in the right environment. Some of us are trapped in a tank that has cut off our growth. You belong in the ocean of opportunity!

We've all heard of the debate between nature versus nurture. The debate is between whether our environment has the largest impact on our outcome or whether our genetics have the largest impact on our outcome. There have been numerous studies done on nature versus nurture. Some researchers have argued that nurture has the largest impact on a person's makeup and some have argued that nature has the largest impact on a person's makeup. I'm not going to make a scientific claim on whether nature or nurture has the largest impact, but I will make claim that amongst all studies carried out, the environment (nurture) does indeed change people. And I will argue this, the biggest influences in your environment are the people you surround yourself with. Don't let everyone into your life and not everyone needs to know your dreams and aspirations. For many, our dreams and aspirations are fragile, and all it takes is for one naysayer to knock us off our course. The greatest people you can have in your life are the people who will build you up and speak life into you. If you want to win in your fitness game, keep the cheerleaders on your sideline!

"Sticks and stones may break my bones, but words will never hurt me" is the biggest lie. Let's take an extreme example of negativity and its repercussions- verbal abuse. Verbal abuse can destroy your dreams and aspirations as it can fill you with self-doubt and a lack of confidence and self-belief. Verbal abuse will keep you trapped in an environment where nothing can grow. It's at your own expense, and it supports someone who deserves less. Cut out the crap that hurts you and surround yourself with what feeds you.

One thing that I believe is important in adding to the topic of your circle of friends, is the importance of diversity amongst your friends. On the topic of diversity, I'm referring to others with different skill sets, different aspirations, different passions, and yes, I'm even referring to others of different races, worldviews, and even religions. Do you know how much you can learn from someone else who's not just like you? Having diversity in your life allows you to see things from a broader perspective and allows you to expand your knowledge. There's some knowledge that you'll learn only from your friends that have different skill sets, aspirations, and passions. Even at a social level, diversity can enable a greater understanding, care, and empathy for someone who is different than you. But more important than anything, diversity challenges you. If you only hang out with people who look like you, think like you, and dream like you, you are missing out on greater opportunity!

You're the project manager; it's your job to build your environment of success. It's your job to put the right soil in place. It's your job to lay the foundation. It's your job to put the right people in place. Control the climate to assist in your nourishment. Creating your environment for success is one of the most important parts of the process.

Motivation for You: Haters

Don't share your dreams with everybody! Not everyone needs to know your dreams. You have people in your life who don't want to see you succeed. People who are naysayers, people who are doubters, even people who are haters. Because of their insecurities, because they haven't been able to accomplish the goals that you've set out to accomplish, they actually want you to fail. In fact, if you do fail in accomplishing your goals, it makes them feel better that they were unable to accomplish their goals.

I've heard far too many motivational speeches about proving naysayers and haters wrong. I say something different. It's not about proving them wrong. It's about proving yourself right! It's about staying secure in your identity. It's not about taking the negative energy and throwing it back and getting revenge. It's about taking the negative energy, smashing it down beneath your feet, then using it as a stepping-stone to elevate you. Don't even waste your energy trying to prove someone else wrong. If you are spending your time trying to prove someone else wrong, you've allowed someone else's negative opinion to influence you. Spending time trying to prove someone wrong is a distraction. **Vengeance is an action of the distracted.** If you allow someone's negative energy to distract you, that's proof that you are allowing someone else to possess a measure of power over you.

I once heard someone put it like this- If you had $86,400 in your bank account and someone stole $10, would you throw away the remaining $86,390 in hopes of getting back at them? Of course not! Everyday, you are given 86,400 seconds. Don't let 10 seconds of someone's negative energy ruin the other 86,390 seconds. If revenge is your focus, they are winning the battle because you are busy reacting to a distraction. It's not their negative energy that's going to slow you down; it's you wasting time on your reaction.

If someone is talking bad behind your back, it's because they are behind you and they can't keep up with your pace. People will only trash talk behind your back. Don't slow yourself down by turning around to confront them. They are behind you for a reason. Separate yourself from them by making the gap wider. My father was my track coach when I was a kid, and he would always tell me in a race to never look back. Why? The simple movement of looking back at someone will only slow us down. That message always stuck with me. Rise above reproach, leave them further behind, and keep your eyes on the finish line. Beat them!

It's a powerful gift to be able to recognize those that help produce greatness within you and challenge you to run faster. Stay with those runners because they will keep you accountable. The process is about being successful in running your race. Value those friendships and keep them in your corner.

"Stop trying to sit at the table with people who have YOU on the menu. While you are struggling with self-doubt, they're intimidated by your full potential." -Chris Griffin IFBB Pro. You're going to have naysayers, doubters, and haters. Put yourself on the stage for them to watch you. It's time to put yourself in the spotlight! Set yourself on fire for the world to watch you burn! "I will show you how great I am!"

-Chapter 9-
The Life of Discipline

"Don't approach your starting line questioning how fast you can do it. Approach your starting line questioning how consistent of a pace you can maintain."
-Trey Patterson

All of us are in a different place within the process of change and transformation. In Chapter 7, I discussed the importance of discovering what you enjoy. This is crucial for the individual who struggles with finding the motivation to get started in their process and/or is new in their regimen. In this chapter, I'm going to speak to a slightly different audience. I'm going to speak to the individual who may have no problem starting a new regimen but struggles to stay committed long-term, or they just can't really seem to find that breakthrough to take it to the next level.

I've always played competitive sports, from my youth even into my adulthood. Because of this, I've known many guys through the years that have made it into the professional circuit. In my youth, I played club soccer with a couple others that eventually became professional soccer players. When I was a men's physique bodybuilder, I competed with and made friends with many guys that became IFBB professional bodybuilders. Today, with over 10 years of being a full-time fitness trainer, I've had the opportunity to build a relationship with many extremely successful executives, entrepreneurs, and many professional athletes. Amongst all of these athletes, executives, and entrepreneurs whom I will refer to as professionals, there is one undeniable common characteristic amongst all of them. Every single one of them were extremely disciplined. They were disciplined in and outside of their work; they were disciplined on and off the field.

In your personal health and fitness journey, discipline extends beyond just going to the gym even if you don't feel like it. It extends beyond saying no to the foods that aren't productive toward your individual goals. And it extends to all those small disciplines. It may seem insignificant to have the discipline to not go to the grocery store when you're hungry, or time your meals to your workouts for greater productivity during your workout sessions. All the small disciplines you create will make a huge difference. Paying attention to the details is what separates a semi-professional from a professional. It separates the good from the great. It separates the worker from the executive.

While the small disciplines are extremely important, I'm going to discuss what I believe are the three most important disciplines to develop if you want to be successful in your health and fitness journey. And then I'm going to come full circle and give you a practical tool in how to create a more disciplined life. Every professional I've ever known and anyone who was wildly successful in their transformation journey had three disciplines that they thrive on. I believe that if you can master these disciplines, you'll reach greater success- 1.

Consistency 2. Self-Control. 3. Patience. One of the most important parts of the process is about developing these disciplines.

Consistency

Consistency is an important discipline to develop. If the process is defined as "a series of actions or steps taken in order to achieve a particular end"; then, the only way you'll achieve the particular end is through consistency. An entire book can be written on successes that were produced from someone's consistency. The greatest inventions and businesses came from consistent improvements. The greatest transformations came from the consistency in developing and strengthening new habits.

Some people wait to find the motivation with the mindset that motivation is what is going to keep them consistent. There are things that we can do to increase our motivation level, but the reality is, we won't always be at our peak motivation. Motivation will waver and there will even be days where you lack all motivation. It's easy to remain consistent when you have a lot of motivation. The battle is in remaining consistent when the motivation leaves. Discipline is about remaining consistent despite being tired and sick of the grind. Don't strive to produce results through a place of motivation, strive to produce results out of consistent effort. In terms of motivation, quite frankly, I believe that some of the greatest motivation comes from consistency. Consistency yields results. There is almost nothing more motivating than seeing results. There is almost nothing more unmotivating than a setback caused by the lack of consistency. If you are trying to lose weight and through a consistent regimen and routines, you drop two dress sizes in your first six weeks, imagine how much fuel you'll add to your fire!

In the 4-Step Evolution of Change, consistency is how your actions convert into habits. Without consistency, a habit will never form. And through being consistent in your habits, the habits become stronger. This is where the greater outcomes are experienced. Part of the process is in developing the discipline of consistency.

Self-Control

Self-control is an important discipline to develop. All disciplines to be developed become stronger the more that you exercise them, especially the discipline of self-control. In fact, this is Webster's definition of self-control - "restraint exercised over one's own impulses, emotions, or desires."

Recently I had dinner with a good buddy of mine. At dinner, we both ordered the same appetizer. Truthfully I don't remember what it was, but I remember both of us loved it. "Wow, this is good! This is one of the best appetizers I've ever had!" In one instant, while we were both indulging, my friend had a very apparent demeanor change. Then he sat up higher in his chair, pushed the appetizer away from him and claimed that he wasn't hungry. He almost looked bothered by something. I didn't really think much about it at the time, but as the evening continued, it kept coming to remembrance. Later that evening while having casual conversation with him, I asked him what probably seemed like a weird question, but I asked why he pushed the appetizer away at dinner. He said, "I just don't like to overindulge. I'll stop myself when I feel like I'm crossing that line." Seems silly right? That was my initial reaction. However, the more I've thought about his comment, the more I began to realize the power of practicing self-control. **If you can develop the discipline of self-control in one area of your life, you'll develop self-control in every area of your life.** While it may seem over the top to "push the appetizer away," if you struggle with developing self-control in one area of your life, start practicing self-control in other areas of your life. Self-control is the ability to carry out rules or behaviors that you set for yourself and the ability to overcome the temptations or urges that you are faced with. If you can't control your temptations or urges, your temptations or urges can take control of you. We are all controlled by something, whether that is someone else, something else, or ourselves. Having control over yourself gives you the full freedom and permission to succeed.

One of the most detrimental things to your success is a lack of self-control. Apart from the obvious, having a lack of self-control will have a negative influence on behaviors. In a professional realm, having self-control or a lack of self-control will determine success probability. Every single one of us knows someone who has lost their job because they lacked self-control. They acted on impulse and lashed out at their boss. They acted inappropriately with another coworker and acted on their urges. I've known many fitness trainers with talent far greater than mine that have thrown away their jobs and their reputation because of one moment when they lacked self-control. Many have sacrificed great opportunity because of something temporary, of which they later regretted. When urges and temptations form, fight for self-control. The fight is within the mind. Don't do what you feel like doing, do what you know to do. That's the differentiator. Someone else seeks to satisfy an indulgence. But Jack is on a journey to strengthen willpower. Be like Jack. Someone else lives to eat. But Jack eats to live. Be like Jack. Someone eats for pleasure. But Jack eats for purpose. Be like Jack.

Sometimes your goals aren't going to cooperate with your feelings, and sometimes your feelings aren't going to cooperate with your dreams.

What if every day you became mindful of your indulgences and you developed self-control the moment that you realize you've crossed the line and you are now overindulging? If you can't control your indulgences, your indulgences can control you. If discipline is strengthened through consistency, then developing greater discipline in one area of your life will lead to greater discipline in all areas of your life. **Once you recognize that the benefits of a healthy lifestyle outweigh the pleasures that you get from an unhealthy lifestyle, and you can develop the discipline of self-control, then you'll reach greater success.**

Patience

I want those results, and I want those results now! I want success, and I want success now!

"I trained 4 years to run 9 seconds, and people give up when they don't see results in 2 months." - Usain Bolt

There are two people driving the same type of car with the same gas mileage. They both pull up to the starting line, and the gun fires to initiate the start of the race. However, it's not a race for time, it's a race for distance to see who can make it the furthest. They both take off heading in the same direction taking the exact same route. Person A decides to speed going 100 mph the entire time, while only getting 20 miles per gallon. Person B decides to drive the speed limit going 70mph, while getting 24 miles per gallon. Who will make it the furthest distance? Person B.

In the process, the goal is to see how far you can go, not how fast you can get there. Remove time from the equation because the greatest successes take time.

When was the last time that you had an absolutely amazing meal that was made in a microwave? If it was that good, everyone would be eating it. If it was that easy, everyone would be doing it. Nothing that is made quickly and easily is of quality. Sometimes we get anxious to accomplish our goals because of our big ambitions, but the outcome is always better when we embrace the process. In the same way that the best food is produced through patience; the best physiques are developed through patience.

We want to do everything we can to accomplish our goals faster and speed up the process. Why? It's because we live in a fast food, microwave society. We are conditioned to want convenience and quickness. We are conditioned to sprint. And the crazy thing is that convenience and quickness are only going to accelerate in the years to come. Assuming you live in a metropolitan area, today you can order something online and have it shipped to your door by <u>3 p.m. tomorrow</u>. In some cases, you can get same day delivery. We want everything now, and we live in a society where we can get almost everything now. We live in the Amazon generation that has set a new standard for convenience and quickness.

We try something and then we stop because we don't see a quick return. If you could just stay patient a little longer, you could have the solution and you can reach a further destination. Almost everything great took time to build. We are taught to value convenience, not patience with reward. We are taught to value quick and easy, not patience with quality. We are conditioned to sprint, not to run for distance. Now, I understand that I may not be speaking to everyone on this topic. Someone reading this may be seeking those quick, 4-12 week results, because they have that upcoming beach vacation or that upcoming wedding, and that's fine. We all have our short-term goals where we want to see change. I'm speaking to those who are on the on the journey to create a sustainable transformation. The race to success is never a sprint.

We've all heard the phrase, slow and steady wins the race. I'm going to change that verbiage a little as I don't like the verbiage of "slow" and steady. Having patience doesn't equal "slow." And, you can be aggressive in a race yet still have patience. Gradual and steady wins the race! There is a reason why marathon runners don't sprint, walk, sprint, walk. They will cover a greater distance with the gradual and steady approach. In this same fashion, you will reap greater benefit in your health and fitness journey in being gradual and steady. A lot of people struggle reaching their destination and it's because of this sprint, walk mentality. We work hard to achieve results for 12 weeks, then stop. In doing so, we've created a roller coaster of obtaining results and then losing those results. We've created progress, which turns into regress. **Don't approach your starting line questioning how fast you can do it. Approach your starting line questioning how consistent of a pace you can maintain.** Be patient, and in so doing, you'll reach your finish line faster. Patience is a discipline that needs to be developed.

Discipline requires practice. Not every day is the day to win a gold medal. Not every day is the day to set a personal best. I've never met someone who went for their hardest sprint and sustained their pace for a long time. If one of the biggest elements of success is in creating a lifestyle change, then make it your goal to make yourself one percent better everyday. That's doable. Everyday is your opportunity to practice. Professional athletes don't become great by playing a lot of games. They become great through practice. Practice doesn't make perfect, as perfection is never attainable. Practice makes permanent.

The gun has fired; your race has begun. Discipline is the gap between your starting line and your finish line! If you want to reach great success, do everything you can to find discipline and develop that discipline, especially the disciplines of consistency, self-control, and patience. The best views come from the hardest climbs. Discipline is the gap between your vision and your success story!

Motivation for You: The Development of Willpower

Through the years there have been hundreds, maybe even thousands of studies done on the human brain to discover if there is a specific neural pattern, gene, or a specific brain activation that can be a determinant of someone's success probability. Multiple studies have found that a specific demographic of people had more development and activation in a specific part of the brain in what's called the Anterior Mid-Cingulate Cortex. This demographic includes a "successful" demographic of individuals including but not limited to executives, and it was extremely prevalent in athletes. Amongst all studies, researchers found that when the participants were forced into a position where they needed to use "willpower," that the neural activity in this specific part of the brain had a spike. The terminology used by the researchers ranged from what they described as the need to use willpower, grit, tenacity, persistence, and perseverance. The more that this section of the brain is activated, the stronger it becomes. Meaning the more that the participants displayed the use of willpower, grit, tenacity, persistence, and perseverance, there was greater activation in the

Anterior Mid-Cingulate Cortex section of the brain. On the flip side when there was a lack of activation of the Anterior Mid-Cingulate Cortex, researchers suggest that the participants displayed apathy or complacency. Wouldn't you like to know what these participants were forced to do amongst all these studies that required them to use their willpower and essentially strengthen the part of the brain that increases success probability? It was activated when the participants were forced to do things that they didn't like to do.

While it seems very complex, in simplicity, the more that you force yourself to do things that you don't like to do, the more that you activate and strengthen the section of the brain that increases willpower, grit, tenacity, persistence, perseverance. If you are someone that gets frustrated and mad because you struggle controlling your actions, habits, outcomes, even addictions, force yourself to do things that you don't like to do. In fact, if you get frustrated and mad because you struggle with your actions, that's proof that you have desire to change but you just lack the willpower.

So how does forcing yourself to do things that you don't like to do translate? Just like I'd mentioned in the discussion on discipline, if you develop willpower in one area of your life, you'll develop willpower in multiple areas of your life, and this has been proven through neural patterns in the brain. As an example, if you've always struggled to develop willpower over your eating decisions, start forcing yourself to take cold showers, force yourself to lift weights, force yourself to do the form of cardio that is hard for you, force yourself to read, force yourself to jump out of bed the moment the alarm clock sounds, etc. If you want substantial power to control your situation, you've got to do everything you can to develop the power of will!

David Goggins, many refer to as the mentally strongest man in the world said, "The main reason I am as strong as I am, is because everyday I force myself to do all the things that I hate to do. It's my lifestyle to do things I hate. Nobody is born with a lot of willpower, it's developed." It's only when you develop willpower that you will have control over your entire life. **If you always struggle with forcing yourself to do the little things that you don't want to do, you'll struggle severely with cycles of addiction, bad habits, and you will struggle with staying disciplined in your goals.** If you have trouble forcing yourself to do the small things everyday, like brushing your teeth when you wake up, being consistent in taking your daily vitamins or medications, or even just waking up five minutes earlier to make it to work on time everyday, you will struggle severely with controlling the best outcome in your health and fitness journey, and in life. If you lack willpower in the small areas, you will not succeed when faced with a major challenge, roadblock, or temptation when you will really need the willpower. **Discipline is a learned behavior that is created through daily practice of your willpower.** The practice of willpower makes permanent neural changes. Having willpower gives you the freedom to succeed. Where there is no will, there is no way! Where there is a will, you will always find a way!

-Chapter 10-
You're a Diamond

*"Your feelings aren't always going to cooperate with your dreams!
And your dreams will never come to fruition if you are led by your feelings!"*
-Trey Patterson

Have you ever studied how a diamond is formed? There are three factors that are needed for the formation of a diamond: 1. Pressure. 2. Heat. 3. Time.

A true diamond is made 40,000 meters beneath the earth's surface, which means that it must undergo extreme pressure. There is no machine on this earth that can create that kind of pressure. Pressure is what contributes to the structure of the diamond. Having been made 40,000 meters beneath the earth's surface, the diamond will undergo extreme heat. Heat is what refines the diamond. It creates greater purity. The last thing that forms a diamond is time. How much time? Somewhere between 25 million to 4 billion years to form. The longer the process, the more expensive the diamond will become. Time adds value. The formation of a diamond is a long process!

(Diagram: Diamond Formation)

→|← + 🔥 + 🕐 = 💎
(Pressure) (Heat) (Time) (Diamond)

In life? Nobody enjoys feeling pressure, nobody enjoys feeling the heat, but don't rush the process. Did you know that the pressure you are facing in your life is forming you? Did you know the heat you are facing is refining you and making you more pure? Did you know that the time that you are undergoing the pressure and heat is only increasing your value? The process is what makes the diamond strong. The process is what makes us strong!

Don't tell me that you are not strong. Over 75 percent of Americans didn't show up for a workout this week. They clocked out from work and just went home and sat on their couch. If you did show up, you are in the top 25 percent! Don't tell me that you are not strong. You're reading a book right now to become stronger, when the majority of America won't pick up a single book this year. Don't tell me you are not strong. The average fitness New Year's resolutioner only lasts 13 days in their fitness regimen and some of you have been consistent in your regimen for years. You've faced the pressures of life, you've endured your hottest summers, you've stood the test of time! You are nothing but strong!

In fitness? Diamonds are formed when you accept the challenge of the heavier resistance. Diamonds are formed when you embrace the burning of each repetition. Diamonds are formed when you feel like leaving early but you decide to stick it out until the end. You've pushed past the pressures and have kept the motivation. You've embraced the heat and finished each repetition. The process is forming you!

The process should not be comfortable. While some may exercise for health reasons, and less for a change in body composition, I'm specifically speaking to the individual who is seeking those physique results. Possibly the most effective workout plan for you is the workout you are not comfortable with. Do you remember when you tried that new workout? You walked into the workout feeling nervous as you didn't know what to expect. You weren't in your element; you weren't in your comfort zone. But more than likely you pushed yourself far harder because of that nervousness and discomfort. It has been proven that a medium amount of stress/discomfort increases productivity. **Your comfort zone is your dead zone.** Comfort is one of the biggest threats to results.

Part of finding success within the process is learning to challenge and embrace discomfort. There is not much growth in comfort, so seek to create a lifestyle of discomfort. Get comfortable getting uncomfortable. Maybe the reason that you are not yielding the same results from your current regimen is because you've become too comfortable. If you're hitting that plateau, it may be time to shift to something else. In fact, maybe the reason that you lack enjoyment in your exercise regimen is because it's become too repetitive and you've become too complacent. Always try new things. It's easy to stay in comfort, but uncomfortable to create movement. There is a direct correlation between being successful in your fitness journey and being successful in life. In life, you wouldn't be the strong person you are today if it wasn't for all the tough times.

Sometimes there is pain in the process. In your exercise regimen, that pain is the breakthrough. It's the dividing factor of growth versus no growth. It's through the pain from lifting weights that you get the most muscle hypertrophy, which means more potential for muscle growth. If it wasn't for the discomfort felt when running or cycling, you wouldn't improve in your cardiovascular fitness. Arnold Schwarzenegger once said "The last three or four reps is what makes the muscles grow. This area of pain limit divides the champion from someone else who is not a champion. That is what most people lack, having the guts to go in and just say they'll go through the pain no matter what happens."

Pain is the physical symptom of you developing strength. No pain, no gain. Embrace the pains that come with growth. **That tiredness, that pain, that discomfort are all a vital part of the process of getting you to the outcome that you desire and are destined for.**

Taking it a step further, if you can master the art of falling in love with the things that you previously hated but make you better, you will completely change your life for the better. If you can find pleasure in the painful experience, you will completely change your life for the better. If you can teach yourself to love healthy foods and love exercise, you will completely change your life for the better. This shift in your mentality is what will produce new outcomes. Now, it's easier said than done, and it will require time. Like a diamond, it requires heat, pressure, and time. The process is the long transition between the new thoughts and your new outcomes.

One of the most iconic speeches to ever be brought to cinema speaks to this topic. Let's take it back to a movie that was released almost 50 years ago - Rocky!

"The world ain't all sunshine and rainbows. It is a very mean and nasty place and it will beat you to your knees and keep you there permanently if you let it. You, me, or nobody is gonna hit as hard as life. But it ain't how hard you hit; it's about how hard you can get hit, and keep moving forward. How much you can take, and keep moving forward. That's how winning is done. Now, if you know what you're worth, then go out and get what you're worth. But you gotta be willing to take the hit, and not pointing fingers saying you ain't where you are because of him, or her, or anybody. Cowards do that and that ain't you. You're better than that!" -Rocky Balboa

If diamonds are formed from pressure and heat, one of the most important pieces of the process is to develop a pain tolerance. It's not just no pain, no gain. It's more pain, more gain. You wouldn't be the successful person you are today if it weren't for all the times you kept pushing forward when you felt like quitting. Maybe you should get excited about all the tough times you face. Maybe you should get excited about that challenging workout that you are about to face. They are your opportunity. As the saying goes, tough times create tough men. Don't try and avoid pain, embrace it, and tolerate it. Your greatest strength comes from your toughest fights.

As someone who has always had a passion for psychology, I became particularly drawn to the topic of pain tolerance when taking my course to become a certified Health and Wellness Coach. Here's a fun nugget for you to take away. At a physical level, there are two things that help pain tolerance- Visualization and Vocalization. You will develop greater pain tolerance if you can visualize your pain as something else. Here are a few examples. If you can, visualize that the sensation is pleasure not pain, that the sensation is cold not hot. Or if you can, focus on the color blue instead of red, as the mind correlates pain with the color red. These visualizations help with pain tolerance. You will also develop greater pain tolerance through vocalization. This includes grunting, moaning, and shouting. In 2014, a study was done where participants did a cold pressor test to test pain tolerance. It's a simple test where participants will put their hand in an ice bucket and essentially try and keep their hand in as long as they can until the pain is unbearable. The individuals who would shout "ow" or even grunt overall had the greater pain tolerance and were able to keep their hand submerged longer. Shouting is almost described as a pain breakthrough, like a sudden charge of strength. (Petersen, 2014). You can alter your perception of pain. Sometimes you've got to keep visualizing the breakthrough, scream, shout, and let it all out. In doing so, you can break down walls!

Motivation for You: Suck it Up

Tough days will come. There will be days where you are exhausted, tired, and sick of the grind. There will be days where the pressure and heat will feel overwhelming. Even tough seasons will come. There will be times where you are mentally at your tipping point, and you will want to toss in the towel and quit on the process. My question to you is this. What are you going to do in that moment?

Everyone is going to face these challenges. It's not about what kind of challenges you face, it's about your response. Your response will determine your outcome. **You are either one decision away from a breakthrough or one decision away from a setback.** This is what is wrong with our society. Tough times come, so we give up. We've lost our work ethic; we've lost our courage. Our response is to quit when faced with challenges. We live in a society where we want everything the easy way. The process is not easy!

There will be times when you feel like you are doing everything you can to find the motivation but you just can't find it. In times like this, the solution is simple.… Suck it up and do it anyway!

Go to the gym. Go get your healthy food. Go back to work. Go back to the drawing board. Just do it. A seasonal exerciser will never get that dream physique. Perseverance is the mark of a champion. You will only be successful in the process if you have perseverance. Sometimes the answer is "just go." You're not always going to feel like working out. You're not always going to feel like eating the healthier foods. **Your feelings aren't always going to cooperate with your dreams! And your dreams will never come to fruition if you are led by your feelings!** Suck it up and do it anyway, despite how you feel!

You are going to have good days, and you are going to have bad days. There are going to be days when you are too tired to exercise. There are going to be days when you are really busy. There are going to be days when you just don't have the energy. Everything in life has ups and downs. Instead of saying "I just don't have the energy today," change it to, "I may not have much energy, but I'm going to give it all that I can." Instead of saying "I'm just too busy today," change it to, "I'm busy today, but where in my schedule can I make time to fit in my workout?" Perspective is important! Even though the goal is to find what you enjoy, it will not be an enjoyable experience every day. This doesn't mean that you're failing in the process. Even if you make every stride possible to have good days, you are still going to have bad days. But that doesn't mean you should call the day quits. Don't ever stop pushing forward because you could be on the verge of a breakthrough!

Right now, someone is extremely successful in the area of life that you want to be successful in. Whether it's with business or fitness goals, if someone else has accomplished it, then that means it's within your grasp. You deserve to win just as much as they do. So go get what you're worth. If you want it bad enough, there is no reason that you can't get it. Your diamond is awaiting you! How do find that diamond? Embrace the process, keep digging, and don't quit!

-Chapter 11-
Victor/Champion Mentality

*"If you can get a promotion of the mind,
you can get a promotion in every area of your life."*
-Trey Patterson

We haven't even scratched the surface on what the human body is capable of! World records are constantly being broken, ushering us into a new realm of possibility. Historically, humans are only becoming stronger. Humans are only becoming smarter. Humans are only becoming faster. The world record deadlift in 1980 was 892 pounds. In 2020, the world record deadlift was 1105 pounds. That's a 213 pound difference in 40 years. The fastest marathon time in 1920 was 2:33. The fastest marathon time in 2020 was 2:02. That's someone running over 20 percent faster 100 years later. In the 2023 Boston marathon alone, 238 people finished with a time faster than 2:33, beating the marathon world record from 1920. Possibly 10,000+ people have broken the marathon world record of 1920 in the past 100 years. The craziest thing about when a world record is broken, is that multiple people end up breaking that previous world record. **A world record being broken isn't just the expansion of a new possibility. It's the evidence of humanity's expansion of mentality.** When a record is broken, there is a new belief of possibility. Someone was able to expand their mentality beyond the realm of possibility.

So what is mentality? It is the capacity of our thoughts and the capacity of our beliefs. The history of records is simply the history of greater mentalities to greater mentalities. It is the physical expansion of belief.

Over the next three chapters, I'm going to discuss the largest factor in determining success capability. Mentality and Mindset. The mentalities and mindsets of success that I'm about to discuss are designed to expand your way of thinking. Mentality is the ceiling of human capability. **If you can get a promotion of the mind, you can get a promotion in every area of your life.**

The lion is the king of the jungle. It doesn't make sense. The lion doesn't have the best genetics. An elephant is much larger. A cheetah is much faster. Orangutans are much smarter. A bear is much stronger. So, what makes a lion the king? His mentality! When other animals sense a threat, they flee. When lions sense a threat, they charge. They will chase after what they believe they can conquer. In the mind of the lion, they can conquer anything. Mentality is everything! There is a lion within all of us! It's time to rise, shine, conquer, and become the victor!

Victor Mentality

Are you the victim or the victor? I'm going to step on a few toes with this one. First, it's important to understand what a victim mentality is. The victim mentality is created out of a negative circumstance or negative experience that you have had that you perceived to be a roadblock or a failure. As a defense mechanism, you cast blame on an outside circumstance or person for the perceived failure. "Surely I am not responsible for this outcome." Truth is, it takes a measure of humility to admit responsibility. But what if I told you that one of the most freeing things that you can do is to take responsibility? If you think that someone else is responsible for your mishaps and shortcomings, your success then becomes determined by someone else's actions. You will never be free to succeed if you believe that someone possesses that level of power over your destiny. The moment you point the finger in blame, you are allowing them to assume control. You will never succeed to the extent that you are capable of if you are under someone else's control.

No one is handed a perfect circumstance. You may not be able to fix your past, but you can take control of your future. Just because obesity runs in the family, doesn't mean that you must accept that you will be obese as well. Just because you were raised in poverty, doesn't mean you will be poor. You may not have the best genetics, but you can still develop your dream physique. You may have health issues in your family, but that doesn't mean that you will inherit those health issues. You may not have had the best schooling, but you can still get your PhD. While some are handed a more difficult circumstance, the victor always sees the opportunity to be triumphant. The greater the battle, the greater the glory, says the victor. The tougher the circumstance, the stronger I become, says the victor. Not everything that happens in life is positive, but there is a positive in everything. Stop being victim to your circumstance and start allowing your circumstance to make you victorious. Defeat is not a position. Defeat is a mindset! Defeat is the position of the victim.

Think of it in terms of sports. Just because you lost, that doesn't make you a loser. Just because you failed, that doesn't make you a failure. Just because you didn't make your high school basketball team, doesn't mean you can't play in the NBA. Michael Jordan didn't make his high school basketball team but became the greatest basketball player and one of the most inspirational athletes of all time. He didn't allow his circumstance to dictate his outcome. He used a negative circumstance to catapult him into the greatest outcome. Michael Jordan is the picture of a victor.

Today, become that victor and view your circumstance not as an obstacle but as an opportunity, because the victor hungers for opportunity. They see a loss as a learning experience. They see a failure as a growing experience. They see a knockdown as an opportunity to get up and become even stronger. Don't ever feel sorry for yourself. That's victim mentality. Instead of saying "why me?" say "try me!" Don't ever focus on what you don't have, but focus on what you do have. You have so much potential within you, and you will never reach your full potential until you see the potential within you. You will not be defeated by what happens to you. You will be defeated by how you react to what happens to you.

"You can't control what happens to you, but you can control how you respond." (Epictetus, an ancient Greek philosopher)

So how does this apply to your fitness journey? Your attitude with which you approach your workouts, even your attitude with how you approach each rep, will determine the kind of results you get. Your attitude directs your destiny. Your attitude is what will determine your altitude. Physically, some people have better genetics. For some it's much easier to lose weight, for some it's much harder to gain muscle. I've known of several IFBB professional bikini competitors that previously were obese. I've known of several IFBB professional bodybuilders that had an extremely high metabolism where it was a struggle to build muscle.

I'm saying this with tough love, but you've got to own your responsibility for not being as successful as you could be, not only in your fitness journey but in life as well. However, don't dwell on what you could have done; dwell on who you can be. Stop being the victim and blaming your significant other. Stop blaming your trainer. Stop blaming your dietitian. Stop blaming anything and anybody for you not being where you want to be. You are giving your power away! Right now, get your power back! You are in full control over your destiny! Don't accept your destiny, rather lead your destiny! Take the bull by the horns! "No man is free who is not master of himself." (Epictetus) If you can control your mentality you will become victorious. If you can learn how to defeat the victim within you, you'll free the victor within you. With no person or circumstance holding you back, you'll turn from victim to victor.

Champion Mentality

While the champion is only recognized in the victory, it was a long process that led to that recognition. The road to becoming a champion is a long road. In the life of a champion, you never hear about the failures, only the triumphs. However, the failures are the most important part of the process of becoming the champion. Our failures are some of our largest growing opportunities. Failure provides experience. It's where we learn the most about ourselves. It's through our failures that we come to terms with our weaknesses. If you want the greatest self-improvement, recognizing your weaknesses will allow you the chance to strengthen them. Failure is discovery.

One of the largest roadblocks to your success is the fear of failure. Don't be afraid to fail! For many, combating this fear will be your hardest fight. It's not the failures that will hold you back, it's the fear of those failures. The fear of failure will withhold you from trying. If you've never failed, it's because you've never really tried. If you never really try, you'll never really have the potential to succeed. I want you to embrace this mentality - "I am going to fail at some point. I am going to have setbacks. I am going to have to learn some hard lessons. I am going to have to grow into my future successes."

Why have I spent the first two paragraphs on champion mentality talking about failing? There are three things that define the champion. 1. They've learned how to conquer the fear of failure. While most fear adversity and challenge, they thrive in difficulty. They are willing to embrace the challenge. They see failure as opportunity. They would rather embrace the disappointment of a failure, than not try at all. 2. They've learned how to fail successfully. Everyone fails. Champions have learned how to fail forward. They always return after a defeat. They don't accept failure as the outcome. They are focused on a victorious outcome. 3. They don't quit. Failure is inevitable, while victory is a choice. The triumphant outcome that has been envisioned will only come to fruition when you don't quit.

Every fitness journey will have wins and losses. There will be times when you see success, and there will be times when you even fail. The one thing that makes this ride a success, is that you don't quit. The reason that someone became a champion is really simple, they never quit. It doesn't even matter what the circumstance is, it doesn't matter the challenge, it doesn't matter what the situation in the world is. Every champion is focused on the opportunity. Stop focusing on the trials and tests and start focusing on the triumphs. Start focusing on the greater outcome! Your outcome is being stronger, your outcome is being healthier, your outcome is being faster, your outcome is being better. Victory is your outcome!

In fitness, the more resistance you add, the stronger you become. It's the same thing in life. The times when you feel the greater resistance are the times when you develop the most strength. You break the barrier. You develop a stronger character. When shooting a bow, the more you pull the arrow back, the greater the resistance, the more opportunity it has to travel.

It's not about how you get knocked down in life; it's about how you get up. Just like boxing, knockdowns aren't important, staying down is! So many people get so close to their fitness goals, but they give up when they hit a wall. Don't ever stop pushing forward because you could be on the verge of a breakthrough. Enough pressure on that wall will make it come down. **When you feel like quitting, remind yourself why you started. Then just put one foot in front of the other and don't stop moving forward.** Look back only to learn; look forward to succeed. You can't drive the car forward if you're focusing on the rear-view mirror.

Most importantly, don't ever decrease your goal, instead increase your effort. Growth only comes when you step out of your comfort zone. Don't downgrade your dream to fit your reality. Upgrade your mindset to match your capabilities. You are meant for more. This isn't it for you! It's only it if you believe this is it! Wake up every morning and stay true to your goals. I will start tomorrow is the great lie of delay! Tomorrow is never now. It's either "one day" or "day one."

Today, begin who you are meant to be. The biggest fight is the start. When you start and don't stop, you become unbeatable. You will experience a level of success that few have the heart to achieve.

"I've paid my dues, time after time.
I've done my sentence, but committed no crime.
And bad mistakes, I've made a few.
I've had my share of sand kicked in my face but I've come through.
I've taken my bows and my curtain calls.
You brought me fame and fortune and everything that goes with it.
I thank you all.
But it's been no bed of roses, and no pleasure cruise.
I consider it a challenge before the human race and I ain't gonna lose.
We are the champions, my friends.
And we'll keep on fighting till the end."
-Queen

It's impossible to beat the man or woman that never quits! So don't ever quit on your goals!

-Chapter 12-
Humble/Confident/Rich Mentality

"In health, fitness, and in life you will not go far beyond what you perceive you are worth, and you will never outperform the way that you see yourself!"
-Trey Patterson

    Successful people surround themselves with other people who are driven toward success. Like the crop farmer, they create the environment to become successful. Let me tell you who your real friends are! Your real friends are the ones who give you honest feedback. They are the ones who will call you out when you are in the wrong. Most people want to surround themselves with people who will only affirm them. But those individuals aren't going to promote growth. We live in a soft generation where being direct is too harsh. Don't be intimidated by people who will be direct with you. The people in your life who will promote the most growth are those who will speak truth to you. They are the ones who will give you constructive feedback. If feedback is a seed of growth, then humility is the good soil that absorbs the nutrients.

Humble Mentality

In my ten years of being full-time in the fitness industry and through training thousands of clients, generally speaking, I have noticed that the ones who are the most successful are the ones who ask the most questions. It's only through being humble enough to ask questions that you'll gain greater knowledge. If humility is the good soil, then knowledge is the fertilizer of growth. You can ready the soil, you can plant the seeds, and you can do the work, but growth won't happen without knowledge. Knowledge gives you the power to change your situation, power to change your destiny, power to change your life. If you aren't as successful in your health and fitness journey as you feel you should be, you may just lack specific knowledge. If you aren't as successful in any area of your life as you feel you should be, it's simple, you may just lack specific knowledge. The individual that has obtained greater success may just have acquired greater knowledge.

Sometimes it's hard to lay down our pride and admit that we don't have all the answers. Pride creates an inability to have self-awareness. It disallows the opportunity to recognize mistakes. It doesn't receive feedback. And it never asks questions. It is one of the largest roadblocks for self-improvement.

By asking questions you're simply maximizing your potential. When questions come, do you seek out answers from friends who may have the knowledge? When questions come, do you try and discover the answers through books, research and Google searches? When questions come, do you watch YouTube videos to educate yourself? Do you even ask questions? If not, you've got to do everything you can to develop a growth mindset and start asking questions. Questions are the bare necessity for growth.

Be quick to listen; slow to speak. Humility is foundational for self-improvement. If you want a higher position in your company or even a higher position in any area of your life, be humble. You will never level up if you rely on yesterday's abilities! You will never level up if you rely on yesterday's knowledge! **The skillset and the knowledge from your past will not be sufficient for a higher position.** "Fake it until you make it" doesn't work when the test is placed before you and the teacher is watching! If you want to reach the level of growth that you are capable of, you must be humble enough to acknowledge your shortcomings. If you are never willing to admit that you were wrong, you will never receive the tools to make it right. No doubt, growth takes a lot of work. A farmer knows how hard it is to grow crops and how hard it is to keep the soil healthy. You'll keep the soil healthy by staying humble. Humility is power!

Confident Mentality

Think of that one person at your gym that always walks into the gym with their head held high. They've got their headphones on. They're focused. They've got goals in mind. And you know they are about to crush their workout. That's confidence!

I'm going to shoot straight to the best solution for building confidence, then come full circle. There is nothing that is going to build more confidence than exercise. Every time one of my clients lifts a heavier weight or runs a faster speed, I immediately see a greater confidence form physically. No doubt that exercise makes us feel better about our appearance, and when we feel great about our appearance, our confidence becomes greater. But apart from the obvious, if you can develop more confidence in your performance at the gym, you'll develop more confidence in your performance in every area of your life. In the most simplistic sense, the reason that the regular gym goers have so much confidence is because they spend several hours a week standing in front of all the gym mirrors, lifting weights, getting pumps, and seeing the better version of themselves. Think about it, in the pumps, they see the more fit versions of themselves. In the sweat, they see the hard work ethic versions of themselves. In the heavy weights, they see the stronger versions of themselves. The better version of themselves that they see in that mirror then becomes their reality. You'll become the person that you see yourself as. If you want to become the most confident version of you, maybe it's found in the gym. It's in the pumps. It's in the weights. It's on the ellipticals. It's in the sweat. And it's in the mirrors!

Confidence will create greater success in every area of your life. It will allow you to chase down the dream physique that you believe you can obtain. When you see the greater perception of yourself, more confidence comes. Your perception of yourself changes your reality. It's not about pursuing vanity, it's about being the most confident version of yourself that you possibly can be.

Years ago as a young motivational speaker, I would listen to fellow motivational speakers at drug awareness events talk about "the power of pride." We were told that pride makes us stronger, pride makes us successful, pride makes us better. The truth is that pride elicits a false sense of accomplishment and entitlement. Pride elicits a false confidence. The iconic motivational speech before the big football game in every inspirational football movie was designed to produce confidence, not pride. Confidence that you have the tools to deliver the win. Confidence that you have the power. If my life was on the line and

I was in combat, I wouldn't want to fight alongside soldiers with pride, I would want to fight alongside soldiers with confidence. Pride tries to force destiny, while confidence draws on destiny. Pride pushes away, while confidence attracts. I think we can all admit that confidence makes someone physically more attractive, while someone with pride becomes physically more unattractive. Someone with confidence has simply established the greater self-perception. If you have a great perception about yourself, you'll attract greater successes. **Confidence is nature's secret and the law of attraction!**

In life, your perception is your reality! It doesn't matter what an old boss said about you. It doesn't matter what a family member said about you. It doesn't matter what a friend said about you. **The only thing that matters is what you say about you.** The only thing that matters is what you perceive to be true. You will put a cap on your potential the moment you receive what you perceive you deserve. You know when someone walks into the room and has that strong presence? He/she must be rich. He/she must be famous. He/she must be somebody! That's the physical manifestation of confidence! Stop looking at where you are at, and start looking at where you could be. Stop looking at the old you, and start looking at the greater new you. If you can learn to see greatness within you, your confidence will be the aroma that attracts the greater destiny!

Rich Mentality

You will only reach for what you perceive you are worth. If you believe that you are worth something, or have a high perceived value, you'll fight for what you are worth. While confident mentality is a high perception of performance, rich mentality is the high perception of worth. If you don't believe you deserve a promotion in your business, you probably won't request it. In your health journey, if you don't believe that your body is worth good health, you probably won't reach for healthy choices. In fitness, if you don't believe you deserve to have a great physique, you probably won't attempt to obtain it. If you do believe you are strong enough or might be strong enough, you've created a higher realm called possibility. Rich mentality is the perception of high self-worth, whereas poor mentality is the perception of low self-worth. Poor mentality gets offered a sum of money, and says, "Wow, that's a lot of money." Rich mentality gets offered that same amount and says, "Wow, that's not a lot of money." The only difference between the two is the perception of worth!

In the simplest sense of the idea of becoming rich, you don't become rich because you work hard to increase your hourly rate. You become rich because you develop good financial habits. In the fitness realm, you don't develop your dream physique simply because you work hard in the gym. You can bust your tail in the gym and still not be close to where you want to be. You'll create your dream physique because you develop good lifestyle habits.

Rich mentality says, "I'm going to save and invest my money, I'm going to capitalize on my gains." Poor mentality says, "I just got paid, I can afford this." Let's flip this and talk about health and fitness. Poor health mentality says, "I just did my exercise, I can afford to eat this unhealthy food. I burned to earn." Rich health mentality says: "I just did my exercise, I'm going to capitalize on my workout by eating healthy." Rich mentality seeks to increase value! It's the mentality that reaches for the greater worth! **In health, fitness, and in life you will not go far beyond what you perceive that you are worth, and you will never outperform the way that you see yourself!**

How does rich versus poor mentality translate to your personal life? Poor mentality compromises your dreams, goals, and aspirations for a salary. A salary is someone else's perception of your worth. Not to say that a salary is bad, but for many it destroys higher possibilities and diminishes true worth.

This is my question to you- Are you so busy building someone else's dreams that you are neglecting yours? Right now, you may have a million dollar business idea on hold because of your $80k/year salary. Right now, you may have a million dollar invention on hold because of your $30/hour job. Right now, you may have a New York Times best selling book on hold because of your paycheck. Stop allowing the convenience of comfort to hold you back from pursuing the riches within you. You must be focused on your own goals if you want to identify your true worth.

In life, every single one of us is meant to do something significant, individual, and great. There is nothing more fulfilling than accomplishing and living out your own dreams and purpose. On a side note, there is nothing more crucial than having the proper work-life balance. As sad as this is, if you were to pass away today, tomorrow your company will start looking for your replacement. And some of us perceive our value based on our company's value of us. Don't look for your worth in someone else who views you as a price tag and replaceable.

If you were on your deathbed and told by a doctor that the only way you could get a cure is to spend everything you had, would you do it? More than likely, yes. Especially if you felt like there was more that you were supposed to accomplish in the world. Especially if you felt like there was more that you were supposed to offer to your family and loved ones. So, you do recognize how much you're worth!

What if you developed the mentality of the rich and could see the greater value of yourself? What if you could recognize that there's no price tag on your dreams and aspirations? You'll attempt to get what you perceive you deserve and are worth. There is never a promise of tomorrow! **I'll start pursuing my dreams tomorrow is the lie of delay!** The bill of regret is more expensive than the price of pursuing your dreams! Don't let the years go by and wonder what could have been! What if I wrote that book? What if I started that business? What if I started that side hustle? In the gym, what if I tried that new workout? What if I tried eating healthier? What if I tried that sport? What if? Don't let those words have power over you! Today, begin who you are meant to be! You are invaluable! Take ahold of your worth and focus on your dreams because your dreams matter!

-Chapter 13-
Progress and Investment Mindset

"Investing in yourself is an investment that will always yield a return. It's the safest investment strategy for your portfolio."
-Trey Patterson

Investment Mindset

In one year from now, you will either be getting paid for the decisions you make today, or you will be paying for those decisions. Truth is, you reap what you sow. **"The best math that you can learn is to calculate the future cost of your current decisions."** -Chris Griffin IFBB Pro

When we think of investments, for most, the first thing that we think of is a financial investment. I'm not writing this section of the book to discuss how you can become rich, as there are many others far more qualified. However, I can say this- The greatest wealth comes from understanding investments. A good investment can offer a 10x,

20x, 100x, even a 1000x return over several decades. They say that a good financial investment should yield a 10 percent return each year. To be investment-minded means to be focused on the long-term reward, not quick return.

    I can honestly say that it wasn't until Covid hit and I was without a job with no income coming in, that I started realizing the importance of financial investment. I was 30 years old when Covid struck, and I did not have much money saved. Once I had this awakening, I started hunting for knowledge on how to create long-term success in the financial realm. I started developing this "investment-mindset" through studying about stocks, cryptocurrency, understanding assets versus liabilities, and studying strategies on how to grow a business. Have you ever really dove deep into studying a new topic, and because you were so focused on this specific topic, you started to view everything through a new lens? For me, this is what happened when I started diving into knowledge on financial investments. Because of this new focus on financial investments, I started viewing everything in my life as investable.

    Through this newly established investment mindset, new financial discipline was created. Again, when you practice a discipline in one area of your life, you'll start to develop that discipline in other areas of your life. Eating the healthier dinner option became an investment in my health. Making the decision to not skip a workout became an investment in my physique. Spending my time pursuing a new certification or new field of research became an investment in my career. Spending 2000+ hours writing a book became an investment in my future. What if you viewed everything in life as an investment? **What you do today has a multiplicative effect.**

Everything is investable because everything has a cost. Watching TV can cost you your time. Getting on social media can cost you your peace of mind. Eating unhealthy foods can cost you your health. Watching the news can cost you your joy. Unhealthy life choices can cost you future medical expenses. What if we shut down social media for a time, and invest that time into mastering a craft? What if we cut back on watching Netflix and invested that time into self-education? I want you to take on a new mindset regarding time. Think of time as something that is investable in the same manner that we view money as investable. Most people live for the moment. It's okay to enjoy your life, buy nice things, and eat the cake. But so many of us overindulge in the temporary for quick satisfaction, and don't leave enough time investing in what could offer a great return. "I want this, and I want it now even if it costs me a lot in the long-run." **The need for the temporary will rob you of your future wealth. The need for the temporary will rob you of your future health.** The biggest thing that I'd like to emphasize in the chapter on investments is this: The overconsumption of the temporary pleasure or high is destroying your wealth and destroying your health. We are so busy overconsuming what we have now, and we are paying little attention to the future cost of those decisions. We are spending too much time doing what's unhealthy when we may not have that much health to give.

We are the credit card generation spending what we don't have. I'm going to refer to this as credit mindset. The idea of credit has changed our mindset on buying and spending. Based upon how much debt the average American has is proof that many are living far beyond their means. How can we understand investments if we are busy spending what we don't have? We buy things that we can't afford, then by next month, we pay the debt. In fact, you can even buy something on credit and wait years to pay it off which only increases the debt. To paint the picture of what I'm talking about from a health perspective, it's like smoking or vaping when we already have poor respiratory health. It will only bury you in further health debt, and for some it will be very hard to get out of. Credit mindset leaves no room for investment mindset.

Prolonged unhealthy choices, from not exercising to overconsuming unhealthy food, will bury you in poor health debt. The deeper you are in it, the harder it will be to get out. Those unhealthy choices will eventually catch up and cost a lot more. You don't want to wait until it's too late to start saving financially for your retirement. You don't want to wait until you develop health issues in your older age to start making healthy life choices. Don't wait until it's too late. Do things today that your future self will thank you for. To be in any measure of debt, financial or health, will rob you of your freedom. If it's an enemy to freedom; it's an enemy to success. Credit mindset is an enemy of success!

During 2022, inflation was at an all time high. Stocks were crashing, cryptocurrency was severely declining, and we were in an economic recession. During this time, a journalist asked Warren Buffet, "What is the greatest investment you can make? Is it certain stocks, real estate, cryptocurrency?" He said, **"The best investment that you can have for most people is investing in your own abilities."** We invest a lot of time as a kid into self-development. But then we graduate high school or college and for most the self-development either slows down or stops altogether. It's almost like society teaches us that self-development is to prepare you for your career, and then once you land that job out of high school or college, there's no more need for self-development.

Investing in getting your real estate license or even that personal trainer certification, as an example, can offer a huge return. Already in a field? Take more classes to increase your knowledge in that field. Adding more certifications/licenses makes you more valuable. Invest in education because knowledge is power. Have a craft? Take the classes to help you improve in your craft. The better the craft, the more it's worth and the more valuable you become. Who knows, improving in your craft may be your next big success opportunity. **Investing in yourself is an investment that will always yield a return. It's the safest investment strategy for your portfolio.**

Isn't it crazy to think that we spend so much time trying to please a boss who may not even like us? We are spending time trying to please him/her, yet we aren't even willing to commit to things that can make us more personally successful. We are investing too much time into making someone else's business successful and pleasing someone else. And we are not investing enough into our own abilities. Investing in yourself and your own abilities is the path to the greater measure of success.

Most people will view beginning an exercise regimen, joining a gym, getting a membership, hiring a trainer, or hiring a dietitian, as a "luxury," not an investment. And in the same standard, view medical expenses as a necessity. Investing in your health is like investing in car insurance except you will have far more "health accidents" than you will car accidents. It's an investment that makes sense. A large percentage of people won't spend a single dollar on health investments (dietitian, nutritionist, trainer, gym membership) which can significantly decrease the likelihood of them developing sickness or injury. Yet, they will spend every single dollar that they have to try and treat a sickness or repair an injury. Most would rather rely on the medical profession to combat sickness, than invest in their health to prevent sickness. In the same manner that we search out investments to increase our wealth, we need to view health and fitness as an investment to increase our life span and overall well-being. Healthy life choices are the preventable cure for most illnesses.

The deeper you drill a well, the better the water quality. If you invest a little more into drilling a deeper well, you can get a better return. Be patient always, because sometimes the greatest measure of increase comes through the wait. The decisions we make today will affect our future, so let's make those healthy choices. We can become healthier. We can become wealthier. We can make our time on earth more comfortable. And we can live longer. What if you lived, in this moment, for your future purpose? What you do today will affect your future. With the investment mindset, you can transform your life in six months. And in the years to come, you can reap both rich wealth and health.

Progress Mindset

Multiple surveys have been taken on people writing books. I was surprised to find out that across the board in all surveys, more than 50 percent of people at some point in their life contemplated writing a fiction or nonfiction book. About 15 percent of people have started writing a book at some point in time. Almost 4 percent of people have finished writing a book. Roughly 1.5 percent of people actually publish a book. With 4 percent of people writing an entire book, and only 1.5 percent publishing it, that means only about 38 percent of people who fully write a book actually publish it. I'm going to make a bold statement. The number one reason that 62 percent of people who write a book don't actually publish it is because of perfectionism. Perfectionism stops publication. Perfectionism stops production. Perfectionism stops progress. Perfectionism makes you believe that the content isn't good enough. Perfectionism is self-doubt. Perfectionism is an enemy of success!

As a society, we would not have all our great inventions, vast knowledge, and amazing scientific breakthroughs if it weren't for someone trying something. We advance because we are always challenging what we previously knew. We would not have progressed this far without someone's effort. Someone put effort into doing something. Then someone else took that someone's previous effort and put their own effort into it to make it better. Just when we think that something has been perfected, someone else makes improvements. Perfection isn't obtainable!

In your health journey, just like writing a book, perfectionism can keep you from starting. It can withhold you from making progress, and it can withhold you from production. That perfectionist mindset will even pull some away from going to the gym or even getting started. If you've ever made the statements, "I just don't know what I'm doing in the gym. I'm not confident enough to workout by myself. Or, I just don't want to get injured." These statements may have been derived from a perfectionist mindset. If you're one of the many that has made these statements to yourself, I want to build up your confidence with this. In my 10 years of being a full-time trainer, I've watched hundreds of thousands of people workout, and some days when training group classes, I've personally trained over 200 people in a single day. I spend more time in a gym than most do at their full-time jobs. Amongst all those, I've seen very few injuries before my eyes and easily 80 percent of them got injured because they were trying to push their weight limit or speed limit. The point is, it's extremely rare to see someone get injured, especially when they are exercising with caution. If I look around at the gym at any given time, I'd say at least 75 percent of people are doing their exercise with imperfection. Your exercise regimen, routine, and form, does not need to be perfect! Despite imperfection, every single person in that gym is making a positive impact on their health and physique. Every single one of them are making an effort. Effort breeds progress.

There will always be room for improvement, so just keep practicing. Practice makes permanent progress. Just keep making an effort and breakthrough will come. Movement is better than no movement, so stop worrying about injuring yourself. **Your fear of what could happen may be holding you back from what you could be!** Fear of driving will keep you from getting to your destination. We all started driving training somewhere. Your driving skills don't need to be perfect, so don't doubt yourself and don't be afraid to make an effort!

I want to emphasize one statement- the goal should always be progress not perfection. The goal should be to develop a progress mindset. Truth is you are going to have knockdowns. Knockdowns are a part of the process. If you fall, fall forward. If you fail, fail forward. The most important thing is that you get up and keep moving forward. The fact that you are even reading a book about transformation already proves that you are part of the minority that's hungry for progress. The fact that you've already started making changes is proof that you are making progress. Don't doubt yourself and your capabilities! Nobody said that the process is easy. In such a short duration of time, you might not see much of an initial reward, but if you keep making effort, one day you'll look back and recognize how much you've produced. If you just keep pushing forward, one day you'll look back and see the distance traveled and the progress made.

-Chapter 14-
The Triad of Success Explained

"After 10 years of being full-time in the fitness industry, it's finally dawned on me. We have an ineffective product!"
-Trey Patterson

Upon entering the second half of The Sustained Fitness Transformation where we will discuss practical ways to create success in your health and fitness journey, let's take a moment to recap the first half of this book.

Diet Culture has created a short-term perception of change and transformation that is a threat to sustainable change and transformation. Transformation is a process and the process is the most important part of the journey. Transformation begins within the mind, making it vital to have the proper mentalities and mindsets. New thoughts create a new belief system which influence our actions. When these actions are created and continued, eventually these actions form new habits. These habits produce new outcomes and changes the identity.

Now that we've discussed how transformation takes place, it's time to discuss the keys to success in your health and fitness journey.

Together, we will uncover all the practical knowledge to deliver results and how to identify the proper diet, exercise regimen, and medical roadblocks. We will address all of our largest societal and personal roadblocks such as inactivity, our largest distractions, and body dysmorphia. And we will learn how to create the most beneficial goals through our own self-evaluation, and create greater motivation to pursue those goals. Let's go!

The Great Dilemma

"Happy New Year! My New Year's resolution is to start exercising again! This is going to be my year to be the fittest and healthiest version of me!"

Fitness is the first place that the majority turns to in the pursuit of their physique goals. Most people have clear goals when they join a big box gym or boutique gym, whether those goals are weight loss, better health, building muscle, etc. Isn't joining a gym the first thing that we are supposed to do when we develop our goals? When they join, even within high end boutique gyms, they are left with little to no direction on how to accomplish those goals. Many who join experience little to no results. For many, after two months of hard work and only losing four pounds, they would get discouraged and call it quits. There is no one there to offer the guidance to make the client successful. In the fitness realm, all that we have been offering our clients is a product. The clients are then sold the product with the hope of accomplishing their goals. A large percentage of those people that sign up don't even enjoy exercise. How effective can that be? For all of my clients that were seeing results, when I asked them what they were doing, it would become apparent that they were doing something else outside of their fitness regimen. Most of the time, they were either on some form of diet or working with a physician. **After 10 years of being full-time in the fitness industry, it's finally dawned on me. We have an ineffective product!**

We have an ineffective product that isn't delivering the results that people join their gym to achieve. We are busy trying to sell our gym as being cooler than the gym down the street. For many gyms, cool has become the main standard for building a successful gym or building a successful product. Sure, cool can be fun but there's got to be more to the product than an experience. Gyms are selling their workouts like beer companies are selling their beer. They put all their focus and money into the marketing. So many of these well-known beer companies simply compete to have the coolest looking can, the best brand, while not enhancing the actual ingredients within that can. Gyms are trying to create a better appearance but using the same workouts and format as the other gyms. It's become a competition of who's got the coolest can.

We are also trying to sell our gym as being the newest and most effective fitness trend. While we do have revolutionary fitness discoveries, there has never been a revolutionary trend that completely changed the fitness industry. All fitness trends were created off of a prior trend. There is no specific fitness machine that is far superior to another fitness machine. There is no boutique gym that is far superior to another boutique gym. Some of these trends include being the gym that is "backed by science" to deliver the most effective workout. Or being that fitness application that offers the highest level of convenience as it offers a workout that you can do in your living room on your own accord. Side note, convenience doesn't always mean increased productivity. It's not that these fitness trends won't work. They will only work if you do the work.

We are missing so many ingredients within our gyms to make the individual with goals successful. In fact, some of these gyms even offer free pizza to entice people to come out, only putting them further from their goals. None of these big box gyms and boutique gyms give the clients all the ingredients to success. In most cases, the only way that you're going to be educated in all the aspects to produce success in your fitness journey, is if you pay an arm and a leg for an experienced personal trainer.

Over the next five chapters, I'm going to share the ingredients needed to be successful in your fitness journey. There are three elements to being successful in your fitness journey. I call these three elements the Triad of Success. If you can understand the Triad, and implement the Triad into your life, you will be successful in your fitness journey. There is also a progression within the Triad, and I list them in order of the progression- 1. Exercise 2. Diet 3. Medical Health. With exercise, we must understand aerobic and anaerobic training. With diet, we must understand resting metabolic rate (RMR) and macros, blood type dieting, and food sensitivities/allergies. With medical health, we must understand insulin levels, hormones, and gut health. All of this information is based on the newest research and development within the health space. Here is a diagram of the Triad of Success that I will be explaining in depth over the next five chapters.

(Diagram: Triad of Success)

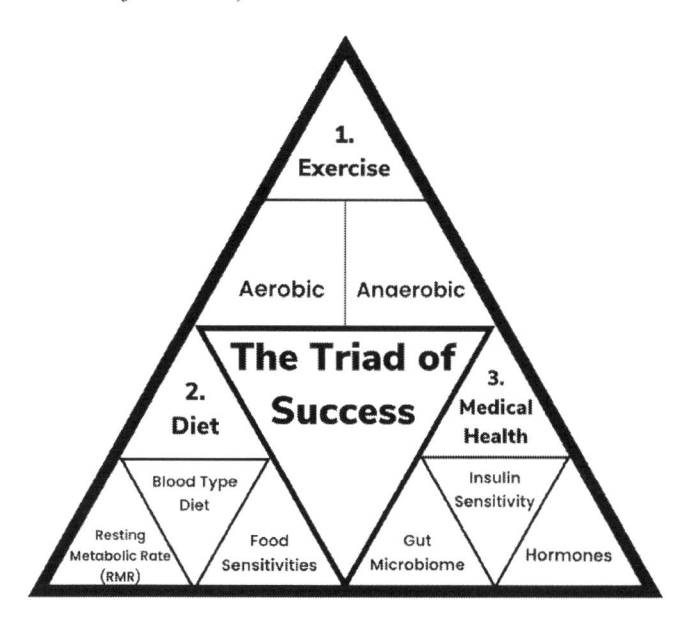

```
                    1.
                 Exercise

            Aerobic | Anaerobic

       2.    The Triad of    3.
      Diet    Success    Medical
                          Health

      Blood Type        Insulin
         Diet          Sensitivity
  Resting      Food      Gut
 Metabolic  Sensitivities Microbiome  Hormones
 Rate (RMR)
```

  There is a powerful synergy between having the proper diet and having the proper exercise regimen. But unfortunately, dietitians today act threatened by fitness trainers and fitness trainers act threatened by dietitians, as if it's a competition. When it comes to general weight loss, there is nothing more important than diet. When it comes to toning and physique development, there is nothing more important than exercise. Another key element is medical health. God forbid you tell a fitness trainer that you are seeing a physician to assist you in your physique goals. However, it is absolutely important to understand that there may be medical reasons why you are not getting the results that you expect. I've given recommendations to many of my clients to see a physician regarding certain conditions. Many of my female clients get diagnosed with thyroid issues, a lot of my male clients get diagnosed with low testosterone, and some of my male and female clients get diagnosed with diabetes or pre-diabetes. These medical issues, to name a few, will have a very dramatic effect on an individual's physique. And these are just a few of the medical issues that are blocking my clients from getting results.

When talking to my clients about their goals, I follow the progression of the Triad with my clients. Upon starting with a new client, my first goal is to create an exercise regimen for them based on their goals. This is the reason most of my clients come to me. They want to take their fitness journey to the next level and become more educated on fitness, or they are struggling to break through a plateau. Let's talk about exercise and why I've placed it as the first element of the Triad. Most that approach me, probably 90 percent that inquire, have some degree of a weight loss/body fat reduction goal. The reason that exercise is first in the Triad is because it's through exercise that new patterns/habits are created, and discipline is created. Not to say that it can't happen, but I have met very few who were enthusiastic about dieting without first being enthusiastic about exercise. Exercise is central to developing new disciplines. Once the discipline is created and someone starts shifting into a healthy lifestyle with an exercise regimen and they recognize the benefits of this healthy change, then we will discuss diet in depth. If they've developed discipline in their exercise regimen, and they've started recognizing the benefits from a healthy lifestyle, they'll be more inclined to be watchful of their diet. Especially if they feel like they've maxed out on the results they've received from their exercise regimen, and are truly serious about reaching greater success.

Exercise

(Diagram: Exercise)

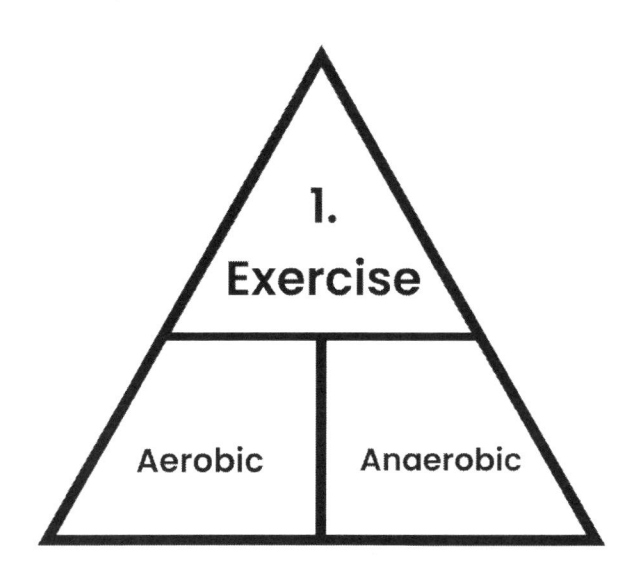

Exercise is the most important element in physique development. Let's take a step back to the basics. We have two forms of exercise that are important to understand- aerobic exercise and anaerobic exercise. They both have different effects on the physique. And it's important for everyone of all physique goals to incorporate both aerobic and anaerobic exercise as there are many health benefits to both. Based on physique goals, you should place more emphasis on either aerobic or anaerobic exercise. I'm not going to spend too much time discussing the science behind the differences of both, but with aerobic and anaerobic exercise, the body uses a different means to produce and exert energy.

Aerobic exercise is any form of exercise that produces a consistent and elevated heart rate. While many forms of exercise can be both aerobic and anaerobic, the main forms of exercise that fall into the category of aerobic exercise are running, cycling, swimming, hiking, and anything similar. Aerobic exercise will allow for a more prolonged exercise session that leads to higher caloric expenditure. For example, this could be 2 1/2 hours of cycling. You'll likely burn more calories within those 2 1/2 hours on a bike than you will in one hour of anaerobic exercising. For someone who is at least 80 pounds overweight or has a body fat percentage greater than 50 percent, I would recommend placing more focus on the aerobic exercise. The only downside to prolonged aerobic sessions is that the over expenditure of calories can lead to catabolism, which means that your body may break down not just fat deposits, but muscle tissue as well. Prolonged aerobic sessions will lead to muscle loss. Muscle loss will reduce the number on the scale, but it's not the target weight to lose. Again, this is why I'm not an advocate for the general weight loss goal.

For most people, at least 80 percent, I would recommend placing more focus on anaerobic exercise. This includes your weight training, high intensity interval training (HIIT), circuit training, plyometrics, or something similar. Typically you'll burn more calories in an hour of anaerobic exercise, especially if you are doing a high intensity interval style of training, than you would in an hour session of aerobic exercise (running, cycling, etc). Weight training, defined as resistance training or strength training, is vital for building muscle tissue. Anyone with a goal of building muscle and gaining weight, should undeniably place the most focus on weight training. It's still important for someone with a weight loss/body fat reduction goal to incorporate weight training as a higher muscle index does increase metabolic rate.

To my aging clients, it is important to increase the frequency of weight training in their regimen as there are many factors that will lead to a decrease in muscle index as we age. High intensity interval training (HIIT), which are short bursts of a high energy utilization followed by recovery, is king for a high caloric expenditure during the session. HIIT training is extremely beneficial to the individual with any form of weight loss/body fat reduction goal as it leads to an elevated metabolic rate after the completion of the exercise. And, you'll more than likely burn more calories in an hour long HIIT session than you will with any other form of exercise.

An experienced personal trainer should be able to identify why a client is unable to break through their plateau and set them on the course for success in their fitness regimen. As mentioned previously, once I recognize that a client is truly determined to change their actions and habits, I then address diet in depth. In a lot of ways, diet is the most important factor in the success of reaching a body composition goal, especially for my onboarding clients, as most of them come to me with more exercise knowledge than diet knowledge. **If your goal is to lose weight, diet is the most important factor.** You can lose weight with diet only, but it's very unlikely that you will have substantial benefit in a weight loss journey with exercise only. **You cannot outwork a bad diet.** I've had several clients come to me through the years with the confession that they workout seven days a week, sometimes even workout two times per day, and they can't seem to understand why they aren't losing weight or building the physique they desire. When I ask them about their diet, they will admit that they haven't been mindful of their diet. The solution is simple. Stop overtraining. Your body needs recovery. More is not always better. Turn your focus to diet.

When I got bit by the fitness bug at 19 years old, I wanted to become a bodybuilder. After two years of spending two hours a day in the gym, six times per week, without adjusting my diet, I only gained about 10 pounds, and most of that I gained within my first year. As someone who was a "hard gainer" in his teens, it was brought to my attention that I wasn't eating enough calories and my body demanded a lot of carbs. After increasing my calorie intake roughly 1000 calories per day and being on a higher carbohydrate diet, I was able to gain about 20 pounds within just a few months, and it was primarily quality muscle. I discovered that I was undernourishing the muscles that I was training to build. It was simple, I was overtraining, placing too much emphasis on my workout regimen, and not enough focus on my diet. I was under-eating and constantly in a catabolic muscle wasting state because I wasn't supplying my body with a sufficient amount of fuel to support my high metabolism and my training regimen. My overtraining was actually counterproductive to me building muscle. This leads me to the second element of the Triad- Diet.

-Chapter 15-
The Complexity of Diet

"The most beneficial diet is the diet that provides a sufficient amount of the foods that are good for your body while also providing enjoyment."
-Trey Patterson

In the summer of 2017, while working out in a 24-Hour Fitness prepping for a bodybuilding competition at 1 a.m., I spotted a guy by the name of Chris Griffin riding a stationary bike. Chris was an IFBB professional men's physique bodybuilder, and even competed in Mr. Olympia, which is the hardest competition in the world within the pro circuit. I was about four weeks out from my second competition and decided to go pick Chris' brain and get some dieting advice on how to "peak" my body for show day. I asked him what his diet looked like during peak week and if he could give me any tips. He then gave me a very profound piece of advice, and it's advice that I've shared with every competitor that has ever approached me for advice. He said, **"I can't give you advice. And truthfully, I don't want to share what I do because it works for me, but it probably won't work for you.**

Everyone's body is completely unique and different." Then he proceeded to share about all the extreme things that he had seen in the professional circuit in regards to peaking the body. Seven years later, these words don't just resonate with me, but it's become a practice of mine when training every single personal training client. I never conduct the same workout with multiple clients, and I never recommend the same diet. In diet terms, one size fits all doesn't exist.

The second element of the Triad is diet. While exercise is extremely important, as it is central to physique development, probably the most important element of someone's success with the goal of weight loss/body fat reduction is found in diet. A lot of my clients will start seeing some decent results with the exercise regimen itself, but it's not until they start dialing in on their diets that they start seeing dramatic results. While I can't give you a generic one size fits all diet, I've created a diagram to help you discover the proper diet for you.

(Diagram: Diet)

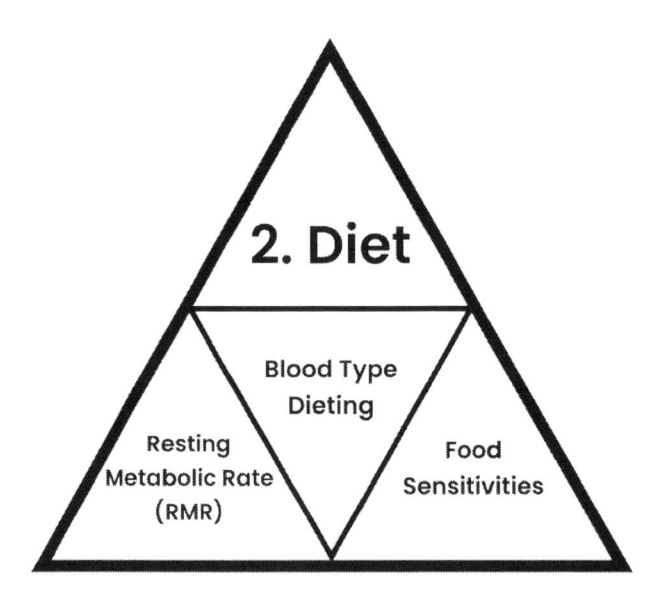

```
                    ▲
                   ╱ ╲
                  ╱   ╲
                 ╱     ╲
                ╱ 2. Diet╲
               ╱         ╲
              ╱───────────╲
             ╱╲   Blood   ╱╲
            ╱  ╲  Type   ╱  ╲
           ╱    ╲Dieting╱    ╲
          ╱Resting╲   ╱  Food ╲
         ╱Metabolic╲ ╱Sensitivities╲
        ╱  Rate    ╲╱             ╲
       ╱  (RMR)                    ╲
      ▔▔▔▔▔▔▔▔▔▔▔▔▔▔▔▔▔▔▔▔▔▔▔▔▔▔▔▔▔
```

Resting Metabolic Rate

Let's break down the diagram of Diet. RMR, which stands for resting metabolic rate, is how many calories your body demands in order to sustain your normal day-to-day functions. Normal day-to-day functions exclude any physical activity that increases heart rate such as exercise, but includes normal activities such as eating, small walks, taking a shower, etc. For most people, a metabolic rate can range from 1,000 calories to 3,000 calories per day, as there is a huge variation from person to person and there are a lot of external factors that can change your metabolic rate from day-to-day. So, if you have a RMR of 1600 calories per day, that means without physical activity, generally speaking you'll need to consume 1600 calories per day to maintain your body weight and provide energy for your normal day to day functions. I do believe it is important to understand your metabolic rate, but I do want to re-emphasize that the calorie deficit approach should not be the main focus of a weight loss journey. There are some situations where a calorie count is important without deficit counting.

As mentioned, there is a wide range in RMR from person to person and a RMR will slightly fluctuate even daily. I've had a few clients that have worked with previous trainers that had them on extreme caloric deficit diets. I'm going to refer to them as starvation diets, and it had a severe negative effect on their metabolism. When talking about calorie consumption, don't starve yourself. It never ends well. If you work with a dietitian, nutritionist, or a trainer, there is no possible way that any dietitian, nutritionist, or trainer should be able to recommend to you an accurate daily caloric consumption count without first knowing your RMR. Not to mention, at a psychological level there is nothing exciting about staying within a calorie consumption count. Again, with that mindset, it will be hard to sustain a lifestyle change.

The most beneficial diet is the diet that provides a sufficient amount of the foods that are good for your body while also providing enjoyment.

There are many self-tests that you can use to track your RMR, and many high-end fitness trackers such as the WHOOP and Oura that track it as well, but the most effective way to get the accurate count is to get tested in a lab for your RMR. Many physicians and dietitians offer these tests, or can point you in the right direction as to where to get these tests taken. Just because someone on the internet said that you should consume 1,400 calories per day for weight loss because it worked for them, doesn't mean you should too.

On the topic of RMR, I also want to discuss macronutrients as well. Just a quick reminder, there are three macronutrients (macros)- fats, carbs, and proteins. Taking a RMR test will not only give you a general understanding of your daily caloric expenditure, but a RMR test should even give you a general idea of how sensitive your body is to the individual macronutrients. For example, my body demands a much higher amount of carbohydrates. Understanding your RMR and macronutrient sensitivity will give you the general idea of which macronutrients to incorporate more of, while not depleting yourself of the other macronutrients like fad diets encourage.

On the topic of metabolic rate, a question that might come to mind is about meal frequency. "Should I eat a few large meals per day, or should I eat several small meals per day? Will meal frequency make a difference in my metabolism?" The answer is not simple, and many arguments have been made for each on its benefits. Assuming that the calorie count is equal, there have been many conflicting arguments. But the truth is, neither method has proven to be far superior to the other one. However, one argument that has been proven is that going for extended periods without eating, also referred to as fasting, does have a negative effect on metabolic rate. When you go for a prolonged period without eating, your metabolism will slow down to preserve the little energy that you have left. And, fasting puts the body into a catabolic/muscle wasting state, and the loss of muscle tissue can have a negative long-term effect on metabolism. So if you are trying to figure out meal frequency, for most, I would recommend leaning toward eating "several small meals" per day.

Since I've brought up the topic of fasting, it's important to discuss intermittent fasting as it's a hot topic. As already stated, for most I do not recommend any form of fasting, intermittent fasting, or fasted cardio because it encourages unnatural eating patterns and can lead to further unnatural and unhealthy eating behaviors. However, there are a few cases where I do recommend fasting and for the ones that I do recommend it to, I do not recommend it as a long-term solution. The main individual that will have significant benefit from intermittent fasting is an individual with gastrointestinal issues or poor/chronic gut health. It will allow a sensitive gut time to rest, and heal, which will help alleviate poor gut symptoms. More people are gaining benefit from intermittent fasting as gut issues are on the rise, but for most it can be harmful, not just from a behavior standpoint, but it can negatively affect resting metabolic rate. The ultimate goal should always be to develop a healthy lifestyle change, not err on the side of a depletion/starvation approach.

If you know your RMR and know it to be slow, do not fear, there are several means to increase metabolic rate. There are many medical issues that I'll address later which can negatively affect metabolism, and through eating a surplus of the right, nutrient dense foods, many of those medical issues can be corrected to ensure a peak metabolism. Here are a few other gems of knowledge to help increase your metabolism efficiency. I would not recommend eating within a couple of hours before going to sleep. Unused energy/food converts into body fat in your sleep. Also, get plenty of sleep. Sleep deprivation can alter key hormones that regulate your metabolism. Sleep deprivation also has a negative impact on metabolism because of its effect on insulin sensitivity and the altering of glucose metabolism. The topic of hormones and insulin are two topics that will be addressed more in depth in the medical health section of the Triad of Success.

Unlike exercise, diet is very complex and unique to each individual. But luckily, we have so many amazing resources that can simplify the proper diet for you. Just because someone has the same RMR as you and their body responds similarly to specific macronutrients doesn't mean that both of your diets should be the exact same. Now that you know how much to eat, and how frequently to eat, you may be asking the question, "How do we know what to eat?" This leads me to the next aspect of dieting that needs to be understood - dieting for your blood type and food sensitivities/food allergies.

Blood Type Diet

Here is the back story about my discovery of blood type dieting. When I was in my early twenties, I used to have an unhealthy obsession with my appearance. I would study every food label and study the ingredients, vitamins and minerals in all foods consumed. I would take pictures of myself every day to study how my body changed. Because of this obsession and watching how my physique would slightly change day-to-day based on what I ate, I became extremely in tune with my body and how my body responded to certain foods. When I was about 24-25 years old, my father, who is also a health enthusiast, educated me on blood type diets. Once I started researching about blood type diets, which foods are beneficial and which foods are non-beneficial, and because of my obsession to be in tune with my body, blood type dieting immediately proved to be useful for me. Almost every food that I knew was beneficial, was beneficial according to the blood type dieting chart. Almost every food that I knew was toxic, was toxic according to the blood type dieting chart. While experience doesn't equal validity, something was to be said about its accuracy for me.

To give a recommendation of what to eat, I believe that "blood type dieting" is a great foundation to start upon. The science behind blood type diets was created by Peter J. D'Adimo. There are eight different blood types- A+, A-, B+, B-, AB+, AB-, O+ (the most common blood type), and O-. If you've ever done bloodwork with a physician or given blood, they should have your blood type information on file. For many, this can be a simple phone call to a family physician or blood donation center. The idea behind blood type diets is that the body responds differently to foods based on your blood type. Your blood type will determine the chemical response to certain foods, and this is mainly due to deficiencies in all blood types. For example, a large percentage of people who are O+ are deficient in Vitamin B, Vitamin K, and Calcium. Vitamin and mineral deficiencies will impact how the body breaks down food. Because of these deficiencies, each blood type will yield more benefit from a specific diet. The most beneficial diet for someone with type O blood is a diet high in protein from meat and fish sources, while someone with type A blood may be better suited for a vegetarian diet. Once you find out which blood type you are, there are several resources and charts that you can pull from the internet that will tell you which foods are beneficial, neutral, and non-beneficial based on your blood type.

Food Sensitivity

While blood type diets serve as a good foundation to get a general understanding of what foods to incorporate or exclude in your diet, not all individuals with the same blood type will respond the exact same way to all foods. This is where food sensitivity tests and food allergy tests come in handy. These are blood tests that you can take to give you an even more accurate analysis of your blood type. This is the third element of Diet to understand, after RMR and blood type dieting. Everyone has different food sensitivities and different food allergies.

A food sensitivity refers to the adverse response to a certain food, and a food that the body struggles to metabolize efficiently. A food allergy is a food that the body perceives as a threat and fights to destroy. I highly recommend getting both a food sensitivity and food allergy test. These are tests that don't even require an appointment with a dietician or physician. You can buy at-home tests online, or even within major pharmacies or grocery stores. I personally have had a lot of success using EverlyWell at-home tests. EverlyWell has a Food Allergy Test, a Food Sensitivity Test (measures reactivity to 90+ common foods), and a Food Sensitivity Comprehensive Test (measures reactivity to 200+ common foods).

Both tests, Allergy and Sensitivity, are very beneficial for different reasons. If you are more concerned with the physique goal, food sensitivity tests may be more beneficial for you as it will help you identify some of the foods causing weight gain and bloating. For example, even if you don't get sick from consuming gluten, you may still have a sensitivity to gluten leading to adverse effects. A food allergy test is more beneficial to take for your overall health and illness prevention. This test will help you identify the foods that could lead to negative health consequences. These tests will give you the general idea of what foods to avoid, not just based on an allergic reaction, but also those that cause bloating and weight gain and can be the open door to greater health problems.

Understanding blood type dieting, food sensitivities, and food allergies eliminates the dieting mindset. **It's about discovering the foods you love that are healthy for you, and leaning toward those choices in your day-to-day eating regimen.** It simplifies the choices on the food menu. Understanding blood type and food sensitivities can actually be exciting. If you love chicken and it's on the beneficial blood type chart and not on the food sensitivity list, then eat more chicken. I'll make this statement multiple times within this book, but the fitness journey is the great discovery. You'll be successful when you discover what you enjoy. And it's even more exciting when you discover the foods that you enjoy and discover that they are healthy for you. You have to consume a diet that you enjoy, and if not, more than likely you'll rebound. This is another reason why fad diets are outdated and ineffective. It doesn't consider your food preferences. The most important factor within elements 1 and 2, exercise and diet, is in creating new healthy habits and patterns with the exercise regimen and diet, and it's only going to be sustainable if it's enjoyable.

Before I begin talking about the third element of the Triad, medical health, I would like to give a long disclosure. As a trainer and health coach, I will never immediately discuss the medical issues with my clients and give recommendations on what supplements/ medications to talk to a physician about. I won't even really discuss the medical alternatives with my clients until they've had a complete lifestyle change through the development of new routines and habits in their exercise and diet regimen. The only time that I'll discuss the medical with a new client is if they describe symptoms/ailments that could be a sign of a medical condition.

Possibly the most important job of a physician is to diagnose and prescribe. So, when approaching a physician, it's assumed that a medicine, peptide, or drug will be prescribed based upon a medical diagnosis. **Drugs, peptides, and medicines, should never be the first solution to getting results in your physique goals.** If elements 1 and 2 are skipped, and someone relies solely on element 3 (medical) for their results, it can actually lead to severe health consequences. If the first approach is to find the drug to fix the issue, a drug isn't going to fix the root of the issue. It's like putting a band-aid over the problem. It can make things worse long-term, and you can become further dependent upon drugs to cover a progression of a health issue. This is why it's vital to improve exercise and diet habits. A lot of my clients have fixed their thyroid issues, hormone issues, gut issues, insulin issues, just to name a few, simply through the creation of a diet and exercise regimen. I will even argue that a majority of illnesses and chronic disease are linked to unhealthy life choices, such as poor diet, lack of exercise, or frequent smoking. Many doctors will argue that over 80% of illness can be prevented through diet, exercise, and healthy life choices. While it is absolutely impossible to prove that the reason for an illness is due to health choices, there are correlations between some illnesses and health choices. For example, frequent smoking greatly increases the risk of lung cancer. A lot of the time even after a doctor gives a cancer diagnosis, they'll recommend exercise and eating a specific diet as certain foods/ingredients have been proven to increase/decrease the risk of certain cancers. Most sicknesses and autoimmune diseases are the byproduct of poor health.

In a fast-paced society, we are conditioned to want the quick fix pill to make us better rather than investing time into creating a healthier version of us. Because of this quick fix society, less people are talking about preventative health and more people are talking about sickness and cures. We are the reason that our frontline workers are overwhelmed. **The root cause of sickness and disease is poor health choices.** In many sicknesses and diseases, the issue isn't the specific sickness and disease itself. It's the ability for our bodies to fight off disease and sickness due to poor health conditions. And for many, we would rather get sick and rely on medicine to save us. This is the reason that the medical industry thrives while the health industry dies. It's the reason that our physicians are overwhelmed while exercise facilities and dietitians are going out of business.

If you have a severe medical condition, especially one that can potentially be fatal if untreated, then absolutely trust your doctor and take the medicine needed. Again, I'm specifically talking about approaching a physician to assist in your physique goals, and I'm not talking about medical conditions/illness. When it comes to your health, always approach health from a holistic standpoint first. By holistic, I mean seeking natural ways such as correcting a diet or incorporating exercise, to improve health and minor medical conditions. You never want to become dependent on any drug because dependency will steal your freedom. If a client isn't willing to improve their healthy life choices, such as diet and exercise, I will not discuss the medical approach with a client. Disclosure complete.

The third element that I'm going to discuss is medical health. I'm going to spend a little more time on this topic as there may be medical reasons why you may not be successful with your physique goals. A lot of fitness professionals don't like to talk about it, because many hesitate to talk to a physician for assistance with physique goals. There are cases where I have mentioned to clients about seeking a physician to assist in weight loss goals, especially in cases of very unhealthy levels of obesity. In fact, when someone has a very unhealthy level of obesity, the topic shouldn't just be weight loss, but rather weight health. As the medical industry is advancing, there is a pivoting that needs to happen. In fact, we will start hearing the new common term "weight health," rather than weight loss.

There are three aspects of medical health that are important to understand in your health journey, and these three topics are what we will be discussing over the next three chapters- Gut Health, Insulin Sensitivity, and Hormones. In themselves, they all play a major role in weight loss or weight gain. There are going to be other factors such as pre-diagnosed illnesses that are going to affect the physical physique, but I want to draw the most attention to Gut Health, Insulin Sensitivity, and Hormones.

(Diagram: Medical Health)

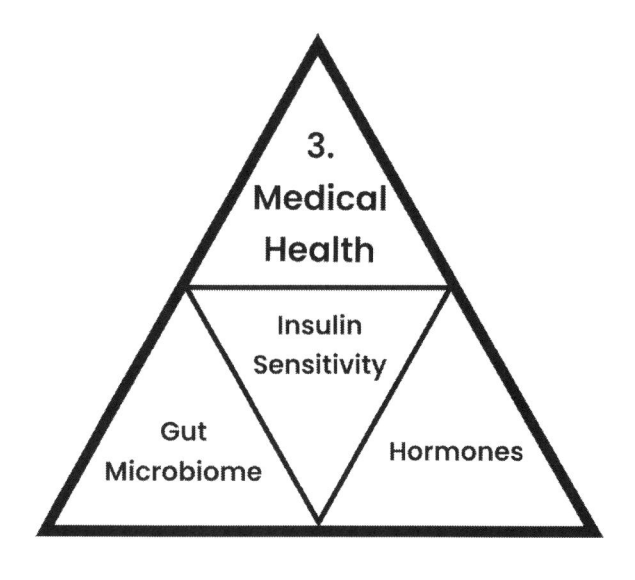

-Chapter 16-
The Gut

"Our environment is changing too rapidly for our bodies, or our gut microbiome, to evolve or adapt."
-Trey Patterson

For most of my adult life, I neglected care for my own health and had unhealthy eating patterns, especially during my years of competing in bodybuilding competitions. In 2022, I developed two autoimmune disorders- Vitiligo and Irritable Bowel Syndrome (IBS). Vitiligo is an autoimmune condition where the body attacks melanin within the skin, leading to white skin patches. These white skin patches formed around my jawline which turned the hair follicles in my beard white in three separate circular patches. Shortly after the development of vitiligo, I started developing severe IBS, leading to progressive and dramatic weight loss over the next year. Upon completion of a meal, I would immediately feel sick and/or develop severe stomach pain. There were even times that the stomach pain was so severe that I would have trouble standing upright, and one of those incidents actually hospitalized me. Little did I know, it was simply the manifestation of a deeper health issue that had been taking place in my body from several years prior.

I'm going to be as vulnerable as possible with you. When I started writing this book, my vision for my book was to create a 150-page fitness motivational book where I would briefly touch on the topics of exercise and diet. Through the development of these two autoimmune conditions, I developed a greater interest in the health and wellness space. Like anyone, I wanted answers to my vitiligo, unhealthy weight loss, and IBS. And unfortunately, every doctor that I visited regarding my health issues was unable to identify a cause, but rather would prescribe a medication to fix the symptoms. Scratching my head, I had questions about the root cause of my health symptoms and those questions demanded answers.

I thought I was young and healthy. As a fitness professional, I felt like I should be the poster child of health. While not all sickness can be prevented as outside circumstances will have an impact, I began the quest to identify greater resources to help us understand our body and health conditions, more accurately. I began to wonder if we can control our health more than we previously thought. In fact, this is the moment that my career took a turn, as my focus went from being a fitness professional to a health professional and after much study, I became certified as a health and wellness coach. One of my goals while studying within the health space was to figure out a why behind sickness, disease, and autoimmune issues to provide a solution for preventative health. Quite frankly, I was just looking for a simple why behind my own health conditions. Unexpectedly, most of the attention turned to studying about gut health.

Why is Gut Health Important?

Gut health is a hot topic not just in the health space but even within the medical community. First, what is the gut? The gut is the gastrointestinal tract, and it mainly refers to the stomach and intestines. It plays a vital role in prevention against sickness and disease. A lot more research about the gut was spurred on after the start of Covid. It is central to our health and wellness, and in fact, 70 percent of our immune system is located in the gut. New discoveries are being made almost daily. In the decades to come, understanding gut health will more than likely be central to the discovery of new medical breakthroughs. The stomach and intestines, the gut, are also responsible for converting food into energy and delivering nutrients into the bloodstream. It is central to metabolic function which is the topic I will be expanding upon more in depth.

Within the gut, we have what's called gut microbiome. Your gut microbiome consists of trillions of microorganisms, or referred to as microbes, that live within your digestive tract. These microbes include bacteria and viruses, and they are crucial to our health. They play a vital role in the body's day-to-day functions as they support immune function, nutrient metabolism, digestion function, and even play a huge role in mood and energy production. If there is an imbalance in gut microbiome, health issues can form such as autoimmune issues, gastrointestinal issues, hormone issues, cognitive decline, and it can even be a precursor to diabetes.

"Your gut bacteria can affect your weight. For example, your microbiome influences how food is digested and absorbed and how dietary fats are stored in the body. An unhealthy gut microbiome can increase inflammatory markers, which may lead to weight gain and metabolic disease. (Nordstoga. 2019).

Apart from the health issues that can form, imbalances in the gut microbiome can be a huge barrier for you obtaining your physique goals, especially with a weight loss/body fat reduction goal.

In 2022, after I was diagnosed with vitiligo and IBS, it was discovered that I had a condition called leaky gut syndrome. Leaky gut is caused by an imbalance in gut microbiome that will compromise the lining of the gut. With leaky gut, unhealthy bacteria and viruses have opportunity to seep through the gut lining and into our bloodstream making us more susceptible to sickness and disease.

"A fast-growing number of pathological conditions, including autoimmune diseases, food intolerances, allergies and sensitivities, have been related to alterations of the intestinal barrier." (Fasano. 2012).

Because of my poor gut health, I lost several pounds of muscle mass and had a huge spike in body fat percentage. My body was not absorbing all the nutrition from the food I was consuming which led to an unknowingly malnourished version of me, hence the weight loss. This lack of nutrition utilization led to a severely disrupted metabolism and these two autoimmune conditions: my vitiligo and IBS. Who would have thought that a gut issue would have such a large impact on not just general health, but the physique as well. Not to mention that I had the largest drop in testosterone levels that I've ever had, which is a key hormone that regulates metabolism.

How Do We Improve our Gut Microbiome?

Our lifestyle choices have a very profound impact on our gut health. Exercise has a positive impact on microbiome. Stress has a negative impact on microbiome. On this same topic, it has been proven that negative emotions/thoughts have a negative impact on microbiome while positive emotions/thoughts have a positive impact on microbiome. Crazy, right? Again, your mind is powerful and even has power over microorganisms living within you. But do you want to know what has the largest impact on gut microbiome? Diet! **As more research comes out, we are only further verifying that we are what we eat!** Foods that are healthy for you will positively affect gut microbiome. Foods that are not healthy for you will negatively affect gut microbiome. And it's not necessarily unhealthy foods that negatively affect gut microbiome, it's what's in the food.

There are several things that we are overconsuming in our society that contribute to a rise in poor gut health. While there is never a one-size-fits-all diet, there are specific foods, or ingredients, that are not healthy for the general population.

The list of unhealthy foods/ingredients is vast and there are a few main culprits behind the societal rise in poor gut health. These include taking various medications and/or antibiotics, consuming sugar, drinking alcohol, and consuming fast food as they all have a poor impression on the gut microbiome. However, above all of those that are mentioned are two foods that we are consuming that are having a devastating effect on our gut health. One of those foods, or I'll say a type of food, that are leading to escalating gut issues is processed foods.

Processed foods take up most of our grocery store aisles today and account for over 70 percent of the traditional western diet, far more than most other developed countries. While not all processed foods are deemed unhealthy, a large percentage of our processed foods come with added food dyes, artificial sweeteners, MSG's, preservatives, and ingredient substitutes. And unfortunately, we have a system that has a low regulation of what ingredients are allowed in our processed foods compared to other countries, especially compared to most European countries. Processed foods may be the leading cause of poor gut health as there is a direct and identifiable correlation between an increase in processed food consumption and poor gut health. **One hundred years ago, we consumed very little processed foods and because it accounts for 70 percent of our western diet today, our environment is changing too rapidly for our bodies, or our gut microbiome, to evolve or adapt.**

Another food that we are consuming in high quantities that is leading to a societal rise in gut issues is gluten. Almost every product made from flour contains gluten such as baked goods, pastas, breads, cereals, etc. More research is coming out that shows how gluten is a major catalyst to poor gut health as gluten is a hard-to-digest protein.

Have you wondered why it seems like suddenly there is a rise in people developing intolerance to gluten? It is only now becoming an issue as our gluten sources, mainly wheat, are harvested and produced differently today compared to 100 years ago. The gluten in food production today is four times more concentrated, and we are consuming at least two times the amount. This means that we are consuming at least eight times the amount of gluten, or a hard-to-digest protein if you will, than we did 100 years ago. Eating gluten triggers dysbiosis which is the imbalance of gut microbiome and it damages the lining of the gut, leading to leaky gut.

If you are someone that has an identifiable gut issue, whether you have been diagnosed with a gastrointestinal disease or have constant acid reflux, diarrhea, burping, gas, or anything similar, then it is extremely important to minimize the consumption of processed foods and gluten. If you are someone that has an identifiable gut issue, there are certain foods that will aggravate your gut issues and in doing so, will be a major roadblock to success in your health and fitness journey. In fact, some of these certain foods are foods that you perceived to be healthy for you. Luckily, we have amazing resources that will help you identify the right foods for you. Wouldn't you like to know what foods are right for your specific body?

The Everlywell Food Sensitivity Comprehensive Test is very beneficial in helping identity foods that are not good for you based on a blood test. However, If I ever have a personal training client communicate that they have gastrointestinal problems, there is another test that I'd recommend before the Everlywell Food Sensitivity Comprehensive Test, and it's the Viome Gut Intelligence Test.

The Viome Gut Intelligence Test is another at home test that can be taken in the comfort of your home. The test will tell you what your gut scores are, whether your gut health is not optimal or average, and it will give you a comprehensive list of over 300 common foods that you should either avoid, minimize, enjoy, or are labeled as a superfood for your body type. The results and food recommendations from the gut intelligence test may be different from the food sensitivity tests, but I find that about 75 percent of the recommended foods are congruent with those of my clients that have taken both tests. As for the 25 percent of foods that are recommended on food sensitivity tests but not the gut intelligence tests, while those foods may be healthy for the body, they are foods that the body may struggle to break down effectively at a microbial level. If you have gastrointestinal issues, your body will not utilize all the nutrition from the healthy foods but can actually create a negative inflammatory response. An example for me includes coffee and a large variety of greens, which I consumed on a regular basis. While these foods have strong nutritional value, for me it was producing negative inflammatory activity leading to worsening gut health and an increase in IBS symptoms. **If you are someone that has an identifiable gut issue, the most important thing that you can do is to fix the gut first!**

The Benefit of These Tests

The Everlywell Food Sensitivity Test and the Viome Gut Intelligence Test changed my life!

Do you remember me mentioning that I had a symptom called leaky gut? Something had to cause it. To help identify what foods could be causing my gut issues I took both the Everlywell Food Sensitivity Comprehensive Test and the Viome Gut Intelligence Test. I was able to identify a few foods that I was consuming on a regular basis that were causing poor gut health, but there was a specific food that I was consuming in large quantities that was having a devastating impact on my gut health. Through taking both the Everlywell Food Sensitivity Comprehensive Test and the Viome Gut Intelligence Test, I was able to identify that my body had an aversion to all gluten, especially wheat. After experimenting with cutting gluten from my diet, and seeing substantial improvement within a month, I decided to take a Celiac screening. I tested positive for Celiac disease. The entire time that I had been consuming this one food that I perceived to be healthy, was actually having the complete opposite effect on me. Gluten was causing my poor weight fluctuations. Gluten was the culprit behind my leaky gut. And gluten was the largest catalyst for me developing vitiligo and IBS. Once I completely eliminated gluten from my diet, within six months I was able to gain my healthy weight back because I no longer had IBS issues. And, I was able to reverse my vitiligo and start restoring the loss of skin pigmentation. And most importantly, I gained my health back.

If you have any gut issues, the most important thing to do is to fix the gut first! If someone breaks an ankle, they'll have to undergo surgery and then they'll go to rehab to strengthen their ankle. Once they finish rehab and the ankle has optimal function, it is then suggested that they continue doing exercises for the ankle to prevent future issues. Think of the food recommendations from the gut intelligence test as surgery and rehab for the gut, and think of food recommendations from food sensitivity tests and blood type diets as the preventative health foods. Someone with poor gut health won't get the maximum benefit and results from consuming foods recommended from the food sensitivity test/blood type diet until the gut is fixed.

To speak directly to those with gut issues, apart from consuming the proper foods to fix the gut issues, I would also recommend regular supplementation of a prebiotic, probiotic, and liver enzyme. In fact, if you ever take the Viome Gut Intelligence Test, Viome also offers a customized probiotic package that I highly recommend. Only then will the metabolism function at its peak at the microbial level. Once gut health is optimal, or if a client doesn't have gut issues to begin with, then I'd recommend that client switch back to a diet based on recommended foods from a food sensitivity test or blood type diet. Once gut issues are resolved, the recommended foods on both tests will be very similar. I do recommend taking both the food sensitivity test and the gut intelligence test every few years, as the body does change and new recommendations will be given. This is evidence that you'll never discover the perfect diet as our diet needs to change as our health changes.

The distinction between this approach to your diet and jumping on a fad diet is that there is no customization in a fad diet. The best part of both of these tests is that they will help you identify the foods that are good for you specifically, help you discover the foods that you enjoy, and will further allow you to lean toward those choices. It will help eliminate the dieting mindset. The discovery of something as simple as an aversion to gluten could dramatically change your health and your physique. The only way that you'll identify the best foods for you specifically are through these two tests or others that are similar.

Autoimmune issues are on a significant increase, and it's because of poor gut health. As a society, we are changing our environment much too fast for our bodies to adapt and its leading to a disruption in the gut. In doing so, it's leading to a sicker version of society. And it's mainly caused by what we are eating. Many medical researchers claim that over 80 percent of illnesses and diseases can be prevented through diet, exercise, and healthy life choices. Poor gut health is even the reason that our bodies are struggling to fight off bacteria and viruses. Once an autoimmune issue forms, it can become genetic making it more likely for a future family member to develop the same issue. We need to start making changes in the foods we consume and fight for an FDA that disallows the sales of certain foods and ingredients. We need health and wellness more than ever before! In a book that is meant to be motivational, encouraging, and positive, it's not my goal to make you afraid, but rather to bring awareness to what is attacking your health. If something is robbing you of your health, it will rob you of the freedom to succeed, not only in your fitness goals but in life as well. Healthy gut, healthy life. Good health is freedom.

-Chapter 17-
Sugar

"In my discussion on medical health, the goal should never be to find a drug to make you lose weight. The goal should be to correct the medical issues that are leading to the weight gain."
-Trey Patterson

Currently, the biggest trend in prescribed weight loss medications is the use of peptides for weight loss, specifically GLP-1 peptides. The main peptides used by physicians for weight loss, are peptides that help the body produce more insulin. Insulin, classified as a hormone, is produced in the pancreas and regulates the amount of glucose, or sugar, within the blood.

When you think of the regulation of glucose or sugar within the blood, you are probably making a mental connection to the word diabetes. And rightfully so as most of these prescribed weight loss peptides were initially designed to help treat diabetes. Some of these prescribed peptides include Liraglutude (Victoza and Saxenda), Semaglutide (Wegovy and Ozympic), and the newest one cleared by the FDA in 2023, Tirzepatide (Mounjara and Zepbound). Once they started seeing the value that these peptides bring in helping diabetics lose weight, it then became the topic of research within the weight loss community. Disclaimer- While I will be discussing why these peptides are effective at helping certain individuals lose weight, I'm not kicking off this chapter to endorse the use of these peptides for weight loss. **In my discussion on medical health, the goal should never be to find a drug to make you lose weight. The goal should be to correct the medical issues that are leading to the weight gain.**

In many cases, someone who has a medical condition, such as diabetes, may need to resort to taking a medication to help manage the medical issue. In the case of using diabetic medications, someone who is not on the spectrum of being diabetic will not gain much benefit from these peptides. In fact, they could potentially have a long-term negative effect on the body. Just because a lot of our Hollywood stars have admitted to the use of these peptides, does not mean you should use them too. There is no one-size-fits-all solution. However, it is important to get an understanding of why they are so effective at helping certain individuals in a weight loss regimen for you to be successful in your health journey and especially a weight loss/body fat reduction regimen.

Back in the 80's up until the early 2000's, most of the weight loss drugs were stimulants. They were extremely unhealthy and extremely addictive, as they were drugs that would significantly increase heart rate. Once physicians started to recognize the importance of insulin and how it affects the physique, the attention turned to studying about diabetic medications and peptides to assist in weight loss. What these specific peptides do is create a natural cell response within the body that triggers the body to produce more insulin. Why does that make them effective in helping a diabetic with weight loss? It's because insulin is in charge of converting food into energy, specifically energy created from sugars and carbohydrates. Insufficient breakdown of energy will lead to body fat gain.

The Struggle of Diabetics

Today, more people than ever before are developing insulin deficiencies and insulin resistance which is reflected on the rise of diagnosed diabetes. In 1990, 4.9 percent of people within the U.S. were diagnosed with being either type 1 or type 2 diabetic. (Harris. 1998). In 2020, 11.3 percent of people within the U.S. were diagnosed with having either type 1 or type 2 diabetes. (Divers. 2020). What makes someone diabetic? Their body is either insulin deficient or insulin resistant. Insulin deficient means that the body doesn't produce enough insulin. Insulin resistant means the body produces insulin, but has an impaired response to insulin. Insulin is important because it is the mechanism to control blood sugar levels. More people are becoming diabetic or pre-diabetic, and there is one main culprit to blame… the overconsumption of sugar!

Let's face it, sugar makes almost everything taste better. Because of this, as a society we are consuming more sugar than ever before. There is a direct correlation between the increase in sugar consumption and cases of diagnosed diabetes. The lack of insulin response or sensitivity in the body will negatively affect cognition. It disrupts body functions including heart functions. It negatively affects your physical physique. And as you probably guessed, it's destructive to your gut health. The overconsumption of sugar will lead to a rise in blood sugar levels, called hyperglycemia. Even if you are not diabetic, you can still get hyperglycemia. Prolonged hyperglycemia, months to years, can lead to a disruption in insulin response. How? Your pancreas is responsible for producing insulin. When the pancreas is working overdrive to create insulin, over time, your pancreas can become desensitized from producing enough insulin. At this level, a doctor may diagnose someone as pre-diabetic. Just like the wear and tear of a car engine, it will affect the performance and over time it will not render the same outcome as it did prior. Simply put, eating excessive amounts of sugars through the years can lead to an individual becoming pre-diabetic and eventually diabetic. If the sugar isn't converted into energy, due to the lack of insulin response, the unused energy will convert into body fat. Someone who is diabetic and not treated with insulin, or a peptide that helps the body secrete insulin, will naturally feel tired and sluggish because of this lack of energy conversion. The topic of insulin is extremely important in understanding weight gain and weight loss. Hence, this is why our breakthrough research in the weight loss field has turned its attention to the effectiveness of diabetic medications like Wegovy, Ozympic, and Mounjara.

Diabetics, who are insulin resistant or insulin deficient are far more likely to become obese than non-diabetics. In 2020, studies showed that about 42 percent of Americans were obese. According to the CDC, 89 percent of people who were diabetic (type 1 or 2) were obese. Many people with type 1 diabetes, need to take a synthetic insulin to make sure the body has proper regulation of blood sugar. Insulin is in charge of converting the carbs/sugars consumed into energy, which then keeps blood sugar in check. The lack of energy conversion and fluctuation of blood sugar levels will lead to body fat gain. If consuming a lot of sugars and carbs can make you gain weight, then why not cut it out all together?

Carbohydrates

Let's talk carbohydrates for a moment. Carbohydrates, or carbs, are one of the three macronutrients alongside fats and protein. Almost all calories come from these three macronutrients. Every macronutrient serves a purpose for the body. Consuming carbs in moderation promotes muscle growth, improves athletic performance, provides energy, and even regulates mood. If you are physically active, it is extremely important to consume optimal levels of carbs. If you've ever depleted yourself of carbs from being on a fad diet, you can attest to how awful you feel when depleted. Carbs convert into sugar within the blood stream, or more specifically, they convert into glucose.

There are two types of carbohydrates–complex carbs and simple carbs. Complex carbs are found in beans, whole grains, potatoes, and vegetables. Simple carbs, also referred to as simple sugars, are found in sports drinks, sodas, fruits, honey, and table sugar. While all carbs, complex carbs included, convert into sugar in the blood stream, simple carbs are fast acting and can have a greater immediate impact on the body. There are four kinds of simple carbs/simple sugars–glucose, fructose, lactose, sucrose. Glucose is the sugar found in honey and some sports drinks, to name a few. Fructose is the sugar found in fruit, some vegetables, and sodas. Lactose is the sugar found in dairy. While most lactose sources aren't that high in sugar and will not have a rapid impact on blood sugar levels, most lactose sources are high in fats which is another macronutrient to be mindful of in a weight loss/body fat reduction journey. And last, we have sucrose. Sucrose comes from table sugar, white and brown sugar, and liquid sugars. All four of these simple sugars convert into glucose in the blood.

Now, before you start telling me that you are going to cut your fruits from your diet, I'm not saying to completely cut carbs as carbs are an important macronutrient, but be careful of the overconsumption of carbs, particularly simple carbs. Again, you don't want to completely neglect simple carbs as they are an important macronutrient and are needed for sufficient bodily functions. Do avoid items high in processed sugars, high fructose corn syrup (found in soda), and especially artificial sweeteners. Artificial sweeteners and high fructose corn syrup have even been linked to various cancers as well. Even though it seems healthier to drink the zero calorie sodas, these sodas use artificial sweeteners. Artificial sweeteners have also been proven to have a dramatic effect on appetite stimulation. Even though you are saving the calories on your drink, it may cause you to consume more calories, which leads me to my next topic. Eating a lot of sugars will create unstable blood sugar levels.

Sugar's Effect on Appetite

There is a psychological aspect to consuming sugar and how it leads to your body demanding more sugar. Similar to an addiction, when your body is depleted, it starts craving more. After each high blood sugar incident, there will be a significant drop in blood sugar referred to as a sugar crash. Psychologically, after a sugar crash when your blood sugar is low, your body says "feed me more." People that are diabetic will tell you that when blood sugar is low, they will feel very weak and drained. Having low blood sugar signals the brain that the body is low on energy and needs to refuel. Now, ghrelin (the hunger hormone) is produced and appetite is stimulated. This is the second reason why eating a lot of sugar is harmful. **Eating sugar stimulates appetite.** Drinking sugary drinks, especially those high in sugar like sodas and sports drinks, stimulates appetite. Obviously when you have an increased appetite, your hunger pains will most likely cause you to consume higher amounts of calories. In its simplest form, a higher consumption of calories will lead to weight gain.

I've got a confession to make, when I go on vacation, I enjoy cheating on my diet. I want to try the local foods, even if they aren't beneficial foods for me and my goals. I want to fully experience another culture when I'm on vacation. In 2022, I went on a cruise with my wife, and my friends Pedram and Mel, where I tracked my weight, before and after the cruise. I gained almost ten pounds on an eight day cruise. I'll admit, some of that was water weight from a high carb diet consumed on the cruise as carbs make your body retain more water. But I did go from seven percent body fat to eleven percent body fat in the span of eight short days. A four percent fluctuation in that short amount of time is drastic. When I'm not on vacation it's pretty uncommon for me to consume sugary drinks, as I typically only drink water, tea, and almond milk. When I went on this cruise, I kept the sugary drinks coming! The specialty sugary drink of the day, "Yeah I'll have another one!" I was having juice for breakfast, sugary drinks in between meals, during dinner, and after dinner. This huge surge in the consumption of sugary drinks led to a surge in appetite. Again, I rarely drink sugary drinks, so I felt a dramatic difference with this substantial increase of sugar intake. My appetite was stimulated because of a rapid drop in blood sugar. On this cruise, I was mindlessly stimulating my own appetite and felt hungry all the time. To make things worse, cruises have 24/7 buffets. Ever wonder why most people gain weight on cruises and at all-inclusive resorts? **The combination of sugary drinks (and alcohol) to stimulate appetite, and unlimited access to food, is the environment for weight gain.**

This knowledge on how sugar stimulates appetite isn't hidden knowledge, but it's knowledge that has been used against us without us knowing it. Have you ever heard of an "aperitivo"? An aperitivo is a sugary alcoholic drink that is served before you eat your meal, popular in Italian culture. What is an aperitivo's purpose? You guessed it! To increase appetite. In the U.S., when you go to a restaurant that has a bar and you're waiting on a table, more than likely they'll ask if you'd like to wait by the bar, or they'll inform you that you can order a drink while you wait. At that steak house- would you like wine while you are waiting? At that Mexican restaurant- would you like a margarita while you are waiting? It's a double win for them! Not only are they gaining more of your business, but they are systematically increasing your appetite.

If you are someone with any health goal, especially a weight loss/body fat reduction goal, eliminate sugary drinks from your house. Those silent but deadly sugary drinks could make up over 50 percent of the sugar that we are consuming as they contain extremely high amounts of sugar. **For many, avoiding those sugary drinks alone, artificial sweetener drinks as well, can make a huge difference in physique, not just in regard to appetite stimulation, but also in the breakdown of energy.** Needless to say, be mindful of the sugary treats in the house like candy, ice cream, and chocolate as well.

Stick with water as water alone has been proven to raise metabolism. Don't like the taste of water? Try brewing it with different teas to give it flavor without adding sugar. Even dairy has sugar in it, which is one of the reasons that I'd recommend unsweetened almond milk for most over cow's milk. If we are not careful, we can add a lot of sugar to our coffee through our creamers and sweeteners. Excess sugar can be sneaking into our diets without us even knowing about it.

Wait, There's More?

Apart from how consuming a lot of sugar leads to weight gain, there are so many negative health effects that sugar has on the body. A large percentage of our major illnesses, diseases, and various forms of cancers, are linked to an overconsumption of sugars. For example, the instability of blood sugar levels can even lead to cognitive decline. Some doctors propose that Alzheimer's/dementia is "type 3 diabetes," as blood sugar plays a major role in cognitive function. If someone you know has Alzheimer's or dementia, be careful of how much sugar they are consuming. If you have a family history of Alzheimer's and dementia, use extra caution in your sugar consumption.

I'm going to discuss this with you from my perspective as a former bodybuilder. Many competitive bodybuilders started taking human growth hormone (HGH) and insulin back in the 1980's. The newest research in the 80's suggested that there was benefit to sugar consumption in bodybuilding as it allowed the muscles to store more glycogen from the increased sugar intake. Glycogen is metabolized fuel for the muscles, which in short can significantly enhance muscle growth. So, bodybuilders started taking insulin and combining it with a carb/sugar surplus as the excess insulin transports the carbs/sugars to the muscle cells effectively. This is the reason why there was a dramatic size difference between bodybuilders during the 70's and bodybuilders during the 90's. In the 90's, bodybuilders were using HGH and insulin combined with more sugars/carbs to create greater size gains. This knowledge on how sugar can assist in muscle growth along with insulin became mainstream information amongst bodybuilders around 2016 as it was addressed in a major men's health magazine. Bodybuilders are consuming more sugars than ever before and many bodybuilders are becoming extremely unhealthy. It's rooted in the extreme need to have an extreme physique. Since 2016, there has been a huge surge in bodybuilders dying of various chronic diseases, illnesses, cancers, and cardiac arrest. I would argue that it has very little to do with steroids or even human growth hormone, but it has more to do with the excessive sugar intake. Cut the sugar. Control the appetite. Keep healthy. Get results.

The moral of the story is, you are what you eat! The largest reason for poor gut health or poor insulin response is our diet. The largest reason for some of our sickness is our diet. The largest reason for some of our heart/cardiac issues is our diet. The largest reason for some of our obesity is our diet. The sad reality is that we live in a society where most want to rely on the medical industry to save us when we get sick, when in fact, possibly a majority of medical issues and illnesses can be prevented through diet and exercise.

Did you know that many cars can be fueled with vegetable oil? It will provide sufficient energy to make it function. However, over time, that vegetable oil will start to clog and eventually ruin the engine. Even when gas prices spike and it might be cheaper to fuel a car with vegetable oil, you wouldn't consider putting vegetable oil in your car because it's too valuable. You wouldn't want to risk destroying a $20k, $40k, or $80k asset. Here's my question to you- How much more valuable are you than your car? How much more valuable is your body? Luckily for us, cars are disposable. You only get one body. What if you switched your mindset on what the purpose of food is? Let the purpose of food be to gain healthy fuel, not pleasure. Let that healthy fuel increase your performance and lifespan.

-Chapter 18-
Hormones

"The unfortunate reality is, for most individuals male and female, the poor eating habits of your youth won't render the same outcome as you age. This is due to a shift in hormones."
-Trey Patterson

Obesity is on the rise within America! Just how much? According to the CDC, "From 2000 to 2020, U.S. obesity prevalence increased from 30.5 percent to 41.9 percent. During the same time, the prevalence of severe obesity increased from 4.7 percent to 9.2 percent." (Liu. 2021). As mentioned in the previous chapter, there is a direct correlation between the increase in diabetes and the increase in obesity. However, there is also a direct correlation between the generational decrease in sufficient hormone production and obesity as well. This isn't new information but it's information that isn't getting the attention it needs. Sufficient hormone production is on a rapid decline. Hormones regulate metabolism, and their decline is one of the leading causes for the rise in obesity.

I'm going to take a moment to speak mainly to the guys on this one. Testosterone, which is the dominant male hormone, also a key hormone within females, is on a sharp decline within our society. **"Average generational testosterone levels in men are declining by more than 1% every year. There has been at least a 20% decline in testosterone production over the past 20 years."** (Andersson. 2007). Guys are producing less testosterone and more estrogen, the female dominant hormone, than ever before. Over 20 percent in 20 years is staggering! At a social level, this should be a major concern as low testosterone will lead to the decline in reproduction, and long-term, a decrease in population.

Apart from the fact that this creates a concern at a social level, insufficient hormone production can lead to many health and even wellness complications. On the wellness side, our hormones regulate mood. Insufficient hormone production can lead to depression. On a side note, with depression, a recent study found that the more time people spend exercising, the better. "People who moderately exercised for 20 minutes a day, five days a week, had a 16 percent lower rate of depressive symptoms and a 43 percent lower risk of major depression compared with those who did not exercise." (McDowell. 2018). Because hormones affect our mood, this could be the key factor behind the lack of motivation and drive to incorporate physical activity. No doubt the lack of motivation and increased depression is going to have a negative effect on health and personal physique.

Hormones possibly play the largest factor in mental illness. Many doctors will link a diagnosed mental illness to a hormonal imbalance. Poor mental health will have a negative impact on your success rate in any area of your life. Possibly the greatest solution to combating poor mental health is frequent exercise. Maybe hiring that personal trainer is a great idea! Some of our behaviors, energy levels, emotions, and our mental health are just a byproduct of our hormones.

I'm going to make a bold statement and a prediction. As humans, we will more than likely exhibit greater genetic changes between the years 2000-2100, than we did in the entire 5,000 years prior to the year 2000. Apart from the obvious self-induced physical alterations that we can financially afford, such as the use of anabolic steroids or other genetically modifying steroids, physique enhancement drugs, Botox, and plastic surgeries, we are exhibiting a huge alteration in genetic makeup. And this alteration in genetic makeup is happening more quickly. There are many reasons for this, but I believe that the shift in genetic makeup is mainly due to a shift in our natural production of hormones.

What's causing this societal shift in hormone production? While there is no single reason, there is a direct correlation to a societal decrease in physical activity. The decrease in physical activity has had a very profound impact on hormone health. Inactivity is a topic that I'll be covering further in this book.

There is also a direct correlation between what we consume and our hormone health. A few of the most common foods that we over-consume that negatively effect hormone health are processed foods, alcohol, and you guessed it.... sugar. Some of the additives, various spices, seasonings, artificial flavors and colors, and preservatives found mainly in microwave meals are negatively affecting our hormone health. Various medications have negative hormonal side effects. In addition, there is a large list of endocrine disrupting chemicals (EDC's), within our environment.

Endocrine Disrupters

The endocrine system is comprised of several different glands within the body that are responsible for producing hormones, including the thyroid, pituitary gland, and the testes. One of the main places where we are exposed to these chemicals is from our drinking water, mainly tap water. Chemicals in contaminated water can negatively affect hormone health and we can ingest these contaminants through unfiltered water. Drinking water from an NSF-certified water filter can help eliminate these EDC's. On the flip side, drinking water from plastic bottles can negatively affect hormone health, as even a minimal amount of plastic consumption is a major EDC.

Another one of the largest sources of EDC's is our fruits and vegetables. It's not the fruits and veggies themselves, it's the pesticides that are sprayed on the growing crops. Pesticides are used to prevent pests and bugs. It is extremely important to wash our fruits and veggies in cool water before consuming as it will help eliminate the pesticides. Your health teacher will appreciate a nicely-washed apple.

And the best for last... There is also a direct correlation between the decline in sufficient hormone production and the overconsumption of foods with added hormones. These added hormones are possibly the strongest EDC's. Synthetic hormones can be consumed through our meat production, especially beef and chicken. Giving hormones to our cows make them twice the weight, produce twice the milk, and worth twice as much. Giving hormones to our chickens make them meatier and produce more eggs. Most farmers are jumping on board, in order to compete and maximize profits. I've always been that medium-rare steak guy, but the more blood, the more potential hormones we are directly ingesting. This is probably the number one reason why many professional dietitians and nutritionists are advising clients to not over-consume many of our meat sources. And some are even advising a vegan diet. It's not that the meat itself is unhealthy, it's what is in our meat that wasn't there 100 years ago.

Combating Poor Hormone Health

I'm going to take a moment to be vulnerable with you. For many years I struggled with low testosterone and poor hormone health. Once I became aware, I developed ways to combat low testosterone naturally. I check my testosterone levels frequently by using Everlywell At-Home Testosterone Test Kits. I've had an underproduction of testosterone and an over-production of estrogen for as long as I can remember. I've always been a big meat eater, especially beef, and I probably averaged drinking three to four cups of whole milk per day. Milk will make you big and strong, right? All of these foods that I was consuming had an adverse effect on my physique by hurting my hormone production. With the desire to boost my hormone health, in 2020, I started making some dramatic changes in my diet. I cut dairy from my diet. I cut back significantly on consuming beef and chicken products, and I even added vegan options to my diet. I've significantly cut back on microwave meals which used to be most of my meals. All these changes brought a sharp increase in my testosterone production. I even had a six week period where I went almost 100 percent vegan and saw an even greater spike in testosterone production. It's not to say that my experience validates a truth as everyone's body responds differently to different foods.

Making an adjustment in one specific area of your life may not create a noticeable change. However, if you are someone with a diagnosed hormonal issue, making several small adjustments in your lifestyle, whether it's the increase in activity or changes in diet, will make a huge difference. Sufficient hormone production is sufficient metabolic function. If you ever go to a lab and take a metabolism test, they typically measure your key hormones.

If inactivity and food production are leading to a decrease in hormone production, then what can we consume that can increase hormone production? Suggested options include leafy green vegetables, fatty fish such as salmon, plant-based milk such as almond milk, oysters and other aphrodisiacs, and nuts such as peanuts and almonds. Healthy fats are good for hormone health. Contrary to all those fad diets that are anti-fat consumption, healthy fats are the most important macronutrient to improve hormone health, which directly increases metabolism. This is why it is important that you are not neglecting any macronutrient as these fad diets suggest. They all serve a specific function.

I do highly encourage many of my clients to regularly take a men's or women's multivitamin as they usually have some ingredients that help with specific gender hormone health. For men, some of the vitamins in supplements that help with hormone health include zinc, garlic, vitamin D, ashwagandha, arginine, saw palmetto, tribulus, and horny goat weed. For females, some of the vitamins in supplements that help with hormone health include vitamin D, vitamin C, vitamin B12, vitamin B6, garlic, ashwagandha, and omega 3's. With the lack of physical activity being a culprit for the decrease in hormone production, increase your workout and exercise frequency. Resistance training and cardio both have a very positive impact on hormone production.

While I don't typically discuss medical alternatives with my clients early on in our training, the topic of hormones is a topic that I usually do discuss pretty early on. After prescribing an exercise regimen to my clients and addressing diet, if they still aren't breaking through that weight loss plateau, I'll then recommend that my clients get their hormones checked either by a doctor or using one of the at-home testosterone test kits. In fact, the most common test that I recommend to my clients is the Everlywell Metabolism Test, as it measures all the key hormones that regulate metabolism. **I've found that more than 50 percent of the time, my client has insufficient hormone production or balance.** For females, they usually discover thyroid complications where their body is not producing enough of the T3 or T4 hormones. The medical term for this is hypothyroidism. While hypothyroidism can affect males, it is much more prevalent in females. The T3 and T4 hormones control energy regulation which affects metabolism.

While possibly the largest hormonal issue preventing weight loss within females is hypothyroidism, in males, it's low testosterone (Low-T). Testosterone is the chief regulator of metabolism and anabolism. While testosterone is the dominant hormone within men, it's still important for a female to have sufficient testosterone production. I'm mainly speaking to the guys on this one, and as a male I can also speak out of experience on this subject. How many times have you heard a guy say, "Once I hit my mid 20's or early 30's, my body started drastically changing"? This is how much of an impact hormones have on our physique. Hormones change as you age and for a male, testosterone production starts to decline in your mid 20's to early 30's. **The unfortunate reality is, for most individuals male and female, the poor eating habits of your youth won't render the same outcome as you age, and this is due to a shift in hormones.** Consuming the same foods that you consumed in your early 20's will have a different effect on your physique in your early 40's and it's due to hormones.

I'm going to dive a little deeper into the topic of hormones because it's crucial to have an understanding of hormones and how they pertain to your success in your physique goals. For many, understanding this topic could be the ingredient you need to break past that plateau you've struggled with. Every client of mine that got diagnosed with a hormone insufficiency and was treated experienced a huge breakthrough in their overall results.

I'm going to disclose some dirt within the bodybuilding community. Have you ever wondered how a bodybuilder who is eating 6,000-8,000 calories per day during their bulk period is still able to maintain their abs? It's simple, anabolic steroids. Don't be fooled, steroids are even extremely common within the female bodybuilding circuit and with male and female fitness modeling as well. What are steroids? Most steroids are synthetic versions of testosterone. That's how they are able to keep their abs while consuming a surplus of calories. Their metabolic response is unnatural because of unnatural levels of hormones. Needless to say, steroids are very unhealthy. These synthetic testosterones shut down the body's ability to naturally produce testosterone. Upon discontinuation of steroids, a post-cycle therapy is required to kick start the natural production of testosterone. If you're wondering how much testosterone some of these top male bodybuilders are pumping into their system, they are pumping 15-20 times more testosterone than the average man is capable of naturally producing. While I'm not advocating the use of steroids, the reason I'm disclosing all this information is because I'm trying to paint a picture as to how significant of an impact hormones make.

I am advocating the importance of taking care of your hormone health. Insufficient hormone production will have the opposite effect on the physique as someone taking steroids. They will lack the ability to build muscle (anabolism), and they will lack the ability to utilize energy (metabolism).

What if I told you that there is one factor that has a greater impact on hormone health that exceeds that of your diet and exercise? Surprisingly there is, and that factor is stress! Truth is, it's hard to make the comparison as diet and especially exercise do have a huge effect on stress levels. Certain foods and the lack of exercise have been linked to increased stress levels, so they all go hand in hand. If you control your stress, you can substantially help your hormone production and hormone balance.

"It's not the situation that's causing your stress, it's your thoughts, and you can change that right here and now. You can choose to be peaceful right here and now. Peace is a choice, and it has nothing to do with what other people do or think." -Gerald G. Jampolsky, MD

Stress

Stress is defined as any type of change that causes physical, emotional, or psychological strain. There are two kinds of stress- acute stress and chronic stress. Acute stress is stress that happens suddenly and usually goes away quickly. It's the quick stress that's caused by slamming on your brakes when in traffic, or being called on by a professor in front of a classroom. Chronic stress is long-term stress. This type of stress can lead to a variety of health issues and is the main form of stress that I'm going to touch on as it has a profound effect on the mind and body. This stress can be caused by an unhappy work environment, long-term financial struggles, family or spousal troubles.

Some emotional symptoms caused by stress include fear, anxiety, hopelessness, and depression. Some physiological symptoms caused by stress are an increased heart rate, high blood pressure, changes in sleep patterns, and changes in immune function. I will argue that beyond the negative physical impact that stress will have on the body, the mental impact is even more substantial.

According to the World Health Organization (WHO), "The world's biggest killer is ischemic heart disease, responsible for 16 percent of the world's total deaths." (Lancet. 2020). While there isn't an accurate way to test for the underlying cause of heart disease, someone can make a strong argument that stress is the leading cause of heart disease based on the physiological effects of stress on heart health.

Stress is the single largest contributor to the lack of sufficient hormone production and proper hormone balance. When under stress, cortisol levels rise. When cortisol levels rise, it will even disrupt insulin response within the body. With the lack of insulin response, your body is no longer able to break down carbohydrates, or glucose, and convert it into energy. This leads to elevated blood sugar levels which leads to weight gain. Chronic stress can be a precursor to diabetes. Apart from elevated cortisol levels, stress disrupts the body's ability to produce testosterone. A large percentage of men who are diagnosed with low testosterone admittedly report having high levels of stress, particularly in their workplace.

Stress can even have a dramatic immediate effect on your physical physique. As I've helped clients prep for bodybuilding, physique, and bikini competitions, one of the biggest charges I give them on competition day is to keep themselves distracted by doing something that they enjoy. Especially on competition day, there is so much stress involved. That stress will have a stronger negative impact on their physique than one meal ever will. Stress can also change our thought processes, actions, and our behaviors. Stress can lead to "stress binge eating" or on the flip side, a lack of appetite with insufficient nutrition. It can elicit unhealthy hobbies such as drug abuse, alcohol abuse, or some similar coping mechanism. And it can create a fitness apathy and a shift in our actions. Actions lead to habits. Habits lead to outcomes. When influenced by stress, we will struggle to control a good outcome.

Stress Management

There is always a solution! Let's talk stress management. I will be giving a holistic approach of five strategies to stress management and why these approaches are effective:

1. Eliminate stressors as much as possible. Now, sometimes it is hard to eliminate stressors as some of our biggest stressors can be work-related or family-related. Family-related stressors unfortunately, are hard stressors to cope with. In most cases it's a stressor that can't be eliminated, only managed. In regards to work-related stress, we are all going to experience stress in some way, shape or form. But, you cannot put a price tag on your health. Giving your best health to your family is more important than giving your best wealth to your family. If the severity of your work-related stress has been causing prolonged physiological changes such as lack of sleep, increase in heart rate, high blood pressure, weight gain, or a weakened immune system, a measure of change is needed in your career for your health's sake. I would like to highlight "prolonged" physiological changes as most of us have probably experienced some of these physiological changes due to

work-related stress. These changes will have a harmful impact on your health and your physique.

2. Exercise regularly. Exercise probably has the most profound impact on stress. Exercise includes any form of physical activity from hiking, cycling, weightlifting, boxing, running, or dancing. Exercise reduces stress-related hormones, mainly cortisol. Exercise also releases endorphins. However, not all physical activity has the same anti-stress benefits. Cardiovascular exercise, such as running and cycling, has been shown to have the greatest benefit with stress reduction. This is due to the greatest release of endorphins. Some would refer to this as the "runners high." Anyone that has ever had a stressful day can attest to how much better they felt after exercise.

3. Eat a healthy diet. First off, a healthy diet always consists of a well-balanced nutritious diet and no depletion of any macronutrient. And it's the right diet for your blood and body type. The most significant foods to avoid are foods that will increase blood sugar levels, those which have refined sugars and artificial sweeteners such as candy, sugary drinks, and other unhealthy carbohydrate sources. The consumption of these foods will lead to similar physiological changes that stress will create. On the flip side, it is very important to consume adequate amounts of healthy fats.

4. Prioritize sleep. Sleep is an absolute necessity for every human being for body function and recovery. Sleep deprivation inhibits brain function, focus, and the ability to carry out general functions. Lack of cognitive function itself is stressful. On the physiological side, a lack of sleep will lead to increased blood pressure which is a component of

stress. And a lack of sleep will inhibit the normal release of hormones and increase cortisol levels. One of the biggest things that we can control that has a negative impact on sleep is television. It overstimulates the mind and disrupts the body's ability to produce melatonin. If you've taken a melatonin supplement and witnessed the benefits from it, watching television before sleep has an unknowingly opposite effect on the body than taking melatonin. Being on a cellphone will have a similar effect. Simply turning off the television and phone for 30 minutes before sleep can help sleep patterns. More importantly than anything, designate a bedtime. Don't let that childhood bedtime ruin your attitude about a bedtime.

5. Make time for meditation and quiet time. We live in such a fast-paced society. There is noise everywhere from the work in front of us, to the television blaring in the background, to cellphones constantly ringing and sending notifications. Quiet time is almost non-existent in our society but is absolutely needed to combat stress. I say this jokingly, but also seriously, people who live out in the countryside with more opportunity for quiet time are more relaxed. Maybe it's an unfair judgement, but you can even hear how less stressed someone from the countryside is than let's say a New Yorker, simply by the way they talk and the tone of their voice. I would argue that the city lifestyle is having a huge negative impact on stress and hormone health. Forcing yourself into meditation and quiet time will disrupt an aggressive lifestyle that's leading to stress. Even just 5-10 minutes a day can help keep stress away.

Stress can have a major negative impact on your transformation. Let's not just manage stress, let's conquer stress. Stop stressing over the small things. **Today is the tomorrow that you were worried about yesterday. You conquered yesterday, you'll conquer today too.** Don't live your life worrying about what could be. Some people spend all their time stressing about what could be, and it's holding them back from being who they are meant to be. **You are living proof that you will survive your toughest days.** You are living proof that you will survive your greatest worries. You are living proof that stress can't defeat you!

-Chapter 19-
The Great Distractions

*"If you don't remove distractions,
those distractions will remove you from your goals."*
-Trey Patterson

Beware! I'm about to address some tough issues, and there will be some tough pills to swallow. These next three chapters may be challenging for some as it promotes lifestyle change. Change is never easy. But if we can search deep, find the will to fight, and examine our surroundings, we may discover a simpler solution for success than anticipated. Let's address the largest society roadblocks to success in your fitness transformation journey!

We live in a time where we have more distractions than ever before. We have a surplus of entertainment on our multiple television screens within our homes. We have unlimited information and media on the phones in our pockets. We have all that the world can offer at our fingertips. There's no such a thing as "I'm bored and there's nothing to do." We have everything to do! While it is great to have unlimited entertainment at our fingertips, if we are not careful with our time, we can develop a distracted lifestyle. While each individual is different, in this chapter I'm going to address the two largest distractions.

The number one reason people give for not exercising is "I don't have enough time." "Time is more valuable than money. You can get more money, but you cannot get more time." -Jim Rohn.

Time is your most valuable asset. Let's first discuss what is consuming our time. When we reflect on what we spend the most time doing, for most, two things will immediately come to mind - working and sleeping. And rightfully so, as these are the two things that consume most of our time. In the U.S., we average 52 hours of sleep per week (roughly 7 1/2 hours per night) and we average 40 hours of work per week. On average, 92 hours of the 168 hours in a week are spent on work and sleep. This is about 55 percent of our time. What are we doing with the other 45 percent, or the other 76 hours of our time? While a lot of time is also spent on accomplishing daily personal tasks, chores, responsibilities, or taking care of children, let's examine some statistics on leisure time activities.

Television

In 2022, the biggest leisure activity for adults in the U.S. was watching television, spending an average of 167 minutes per day. (Krantz-Kent. 2022). According to U.S. Bureau of Labor Statistics, watching television is defined as watching live programming, viewing DVDs, and streaming shows on television sets, computers, and portable devices. This number had a slight increase after the Covid-19 pandemic. Almost everyone watches television, and most are watching more than ever before.

Apart from the fact that the overconsumption of television is the number one distraction, there are many other reasons why it can be a huge roadblock to your success. One thing is obvious, with television consumption comes a decrease in physical activity. It's a couch task. With this decrease in physical activity will come a decrease in motivation levels. There is also a shift in brain activity. Experts refer to watching television as inducing a state of autohypnosis, or self-induced hypnosis, leaving us more vulnerable and susceptible to suggestions. A food ad pops up, giving you a suggestion of being hungry. This is the reason why television is the number one place for food advertisements, especially during prime time. Psychologists dating back to the 50's discovered how powerful television suggestions are on the human psyche; a law was passed in 1958 banning the use of subliminal marketing.

On a side note, because of the shift in brain activity while watching television, I do not recommend eating in front of a television as it can lead to mindless eating behaviors. Could the overconsumption of television be one of the leading factors in the rise in obesity? Sounds crazy, but a strong argument can be made on the negative effects it can have on the physique.

Television itself isn't inherently a roadblock, but the distraction of television could actually be having more of a negative effect on your success than you may realize. What if you took some of that time from viewing television and tuned into programming that has a positive effect? This could be watching motivational fitness videos on YouTube or watching shows that educate you. True story, when I prepped for bodybuilding competitions, for the entire duration of my prep the only thing I watched on television was fitness motivational videos. I would watch fitness documentaries like Pumping Iron, CrossFit competitions on Netflix, quite frankly anything fitness and health related as it created inspiration rather than promoting laziness. I can't ever recall seeing a fast-food commercial come on during a fitness motivational video.

Why? It's because I'm not their target market. By consuming "healthy" content, I wasn't being exposed to "unhealthy" temptations.

What if we turned off the television and spent more time reading? Reading increases brain activity. And there are no food commercials to target you in your vulnerable state of mind. Although we may get hungry while reading, we are less susceptible to suggestions. This goes back to the topic of the power of your environment and recognizing your triggers. For many, our own television screen can be our largest trigger. What you place before your eyes will have a significant impact on your reactions. What if we took it a step further, and turned off the television and spent more time with an outdoor activity? Imagine how profound of an impact it could make if you simply turned off the television for an hour every day and took the dogs on a long walk. If television isn't distracting enough, there is another leisure time activity that is decimating our time... social media.

Social Media

I'm going to refer to social media as the time thief. It's the sneaky distraction. Most of the time, we are well aware of how much time we spend watching television, but social media for many is the distraction that can sneak back in regularly throughout the day. It's easily accessible since most engage in social media on their phones. We get an alert on our phone that someone commented on a post. We open social media to check a notification. Twenty minutes later, we realize we've been wasting time on social media swiping through reels. Many of us can relate. Social media is a smart business that knows how to get your attention. For many, social media can be the gateway to other internet usage such as online shopping, leading to yet another distraction. Many experts suggest that individuals can develop a dependency/addiction to social media similarly to a drug dependency/addiction. It's an addiction to endorphins, an addiction to instant gratification, and it creates the need for constant stimulation.

How much time are we spending on social media? In 2022, roughly 90 percent of people within the U.S. were active on some form of social media. According to the U.S. Bureau of Statistics, "actively" on social media is defined as any unfrozen account within any social media platform from twitter to Instagram, from Reddit to Pinterest, from Youtube to What's App, from Snapchat to LinkedIn, from Tik Tok to MySpace, and it also includes online gaming. "Actively" on social media includes the individual that will check in once every six months. Amongst people who are actively on social media, how much time does the average person spend on social media per day? In 2022, the data suggested roughly 147 minutes per day. (Krantz-Kent. 2022). Since 2012, that number has gone up roughly an hour per person per day. There was a large spike in social media usage after the pandemic, and I believe it was due to more jobs shifting remotely, the Covid quarantine, and the need for more social interaction. In 2022, Facebook Inc alone generated 23 percent of all internet traffic. People are spending more time on social media, and it will soon be the number one leisure time activity as adolescents currently spend far more time on social media than watching television.

Yes, social media does serve as the quickest avenue to obtain information and news. And some of us like to be the first to hear the big news. And to those, I'm going to challenge you with this question. When was the last time that hearing information or news a few hours earlier had a profound positive impact on your life? But boy, can the distractions that social media offer have a profound negative impact on your time!

The media, consisting of social media and watching television, consumes 314 minutes per day, or 5 hours and 14 minutes per day on average. Let's take a conservative approach on how much time the average adult spends on all media consumption, assuming that someone might be on social media while watching television, and let's say that only 4 hours and 30 minutes is spent on these two combined. That's over 31 hours per week that is spent between these two, or roughly 1,616 hours per year to put it in a different perspective. While media can be a tool for your education and advancement, most of it is just stealing our time.

Of course for many, our media provides enjoyment and can be a short and healthy distraction. Our bodies do need the entertainment offered and the opportunity to recharge. My argument is that the overconsumption of our media can create a substantial and noticeable lack of interest in our goals that we'll even blame "not having enough time," as the largest reason for not exercising. **Many of us have created a lifestyle built on the overindulgences of our entertainment and it's killing productivity.** For some, we'll spend as much time consuming media as a full-time job. If your goal is productivity, it's undeniably important to monitor your time. Managing and becoming intentional with your time is an absolute must in order to be successful in any area of your life, especially in your fitness journey. Create a schedule to only watch television within certain time allotments. Be disciplined not to go over on that time. It's easy to watch "one more episode" or to watch "one more reel." Mastering your time is one of the most important aspects of developing a disciplined lifestyle. Something is going to control your time. It will either be you or your distractions. Maybe we aren't really as busy as we think we are. For some of us, "I don't have enough time," is actually "I don't have good time management."

Time Management

I have a client that inspires me greatly with his superior time management. His name is Tim. He's been a client of mine for a few years, and he has also become a great friend. And, he's also become a training partner of mine as I'm currently training for an Ironman triathlon. Tim is the president of an oil and gas company, easily working 60+ hours per week at his job. The first year that I was training him, he had major house issues on one he recently purchased. For over a year he constantly had contractors at his house, constantly moving things in and out of the house. Tearing down walls, ripping up floors, meeting with contractors, working 60+ hours per week, with 1-2 work trips per month. Needless to say, he was busy. Yet, he still managed to train with me 3-4 times per week. Without fail, he set aside time in his calendar to train with me as a priority, and he rarely cancelled. In Tim's words- "You have to make this habit a part of your life or life will get in the way. Everyone has the same amount of hours in a week. You can either make the 4-5 hours of exercise happen, or you can make excuses why it didn't."

For most, self improvement and exercise simply aren't a priority. **Time isn't the issue, priority is.** "I don't have time to exercise," is the adult version of blaming your dog for eating your homework. "I don't have time to exercise" is a euphemism for "exercise is not a priority for me."

Imagine if you just took an hour of that distracted time per day and dedicated it to reading educational books, watching motivational videos, exercising, or even taking it a step further and riding an elliptical while viewing motivational videos. One hour a day, to keep complacency away! One hour a day of reading, watching motivational and educational videos, or exercising is 365 hours in one year. Do you know how much you can change your life in one year by investing 365 hours of your time into self-development? In three years, you could transform your life so dramatically that you will become unrecognizable! This is the essence of a growth mindset! Being aware of your distractions, being intentional with your time, and pursuing the opportunity to learn and grow daily. There is not a more key mindset to your probability of success than a growth mindset.

If you want greater productivity, maximize your time. It starts with awareness of what's stealing your time. While the only two distractions that I have mentioned are television and social media, there are many things that can be a distraction. This is something that may take some time to truly figure out. Take note of how much time you're putting into certain activities. Even if you don't spend that much time watching television or social media, ask yourself if what you are doing is bringing you closer to your goals, or further from your goals. Every person who is extremely successful, whether it's in business or in their fitness journey, is disciplined in their time and doesn't allow distractions to consume their time.

Today, in this moment, you are being handed an opportunity to excel far more than previous generations. How? We have more distractions than ever before, and most are reacting to those distractions. Productive time seems to be decreasing. How you deal with your distractions and how you manage your time is what could separate you from the crowd. You don't have to be distracted! You have time on your hands!

Motivation for You: Finding Focus

"If just for a moment, be willing to lose your connection to the people, places, and things that create the most noise. Your life becomes a masterpiece when you learn to master peace." -Chris Griffin IFBB Pro

Turn down the volume of all the outside noise! If creating new routines is a powerful tool in forming new habits, what if you made it routine to designate short daily time slots to consuming media, whether it's television or social media. There's so much loud noise everywhere that most of us don't even know what quiet sounds like. We spend far too much time reacting to what distracts us, and not enough time being intentional and creating focus.

A big reason that the rich are getting richer, the successful are becoming more successful, and the fit are getting fitter is because fewer are remaining undistracted. The ones who are winning are simply seizing the opportunity. You've got to do everything you can to remove distractions and find your focus! Not having focus is like bowling and not having pins at which to aim. If you don't have a target, if you don't have a focus point, you will never successfully hit your goals. It's time to get focused on your goals!

Where is your focus? When you open up Instagram, what things show up all over your feed? That's what you're focusing on. When you turn on YouTube, what video recommendations does it give you? That's what you're focusing on. Our media today, especially social media is "smart business." They know what gets your attention. There are algorithms in place within social media to feed you with the information that you want to see. It recognizes patterns based on things you like, articles you post, topics that you comment on, to name a few. These algorithms recognize your patterns and will feed you with the information that interests you. You can use this system to your advantage and create attention!

Take a moment and assess your goals. Is the information that you are being fed with bringing you closer to your goals or further away? If your goal is weight loss, you should open Instagram and see a feed full of weight loss testimonies. If your goal is to get rich, you should open up YouTube and see successful entrepreneurs discussing how to become rich. If your goal is to become a bodybuilder, you should open Instagram and see bodybuilders all over your feed.

Here is my point. You can create attention and focus! You can even use your scheduled social media time as a tool for your benefit. **What are you typing into the search engine on Instagram and what are you "liking"? You'll get more of that.** What profiles are you spending the most time viewing and what content do you spend the most time consuming? You'll get more of that. It feeds you the information that you are already consuming.

I'm going to give you practical and relevant advice for the new digital age. Whenever you are feeling motivated with your goals, "like" everything on social media that reflects your goals. "Like" all those motivational posts, "like" all those fitness posts, "like" all those business posts. It's the tiny little actions and disciplines such as "liking" posts that will have a substantial impact on your success. Is it your goal to know what all of your favorite celebrities did today or is it your goal to be the fittest, healthiest version of you? After you start liking all those posts, guess what will happen? You'll get fed more of the content that reflects your goals. And on the days where you are not feeling motivated with your goals and open up social media, you'll be pulled back into your former motivation. In one month from now, your social media feed can look completely different, and that very environment will help usher you into success. No doubt it is a fight to keep your motivation high. Distraction is one of the greatest threats to your motivation. And don't tell me that motivation isn't important. When was the last time that you accomplished something great without first having the motivation to do it.

Can you imagine if you made the decision to make health and fitness your absolute focus, even if just for a few months? In a short time, it could change your life. Like a microscope in biology, if you can make all those small adjustments, it will allow you to see with more detail and precision. In fact, the most complex microscopes require several hundred adjustments. With your goals, detail and precision will reap the benefit. That high resolution of focus will even allow you to increase productivity while being less busy. **If you don't remove distractions, those distractions will remove you from your goals.** Having a goal without focus is simply a dream. Keep your focus, and you'll hit your goals.

-Chapter 20-
Inactivity and Over-Accessibility

*"The digital age of television and entertainment
is keeping us occupied while we sit on the couches of inactivity."*
-Trey Patterson

There are so many options of local gyms and exercise classes that we can join. We have gyms of all shapes and sizes. We have exercise classes for every body type, every personality, and every fitness level. This apparent gold rush of opening another gym and exercise class must mean that we are more active than ever before, correct? While it may appear that the fitness industry is on the rise in terms of engagement, the truth is, physical activity is on a substantial decline.

The Inactive Generation

We, Americans, are the most inactive that we have ever been. How can this be? Let's start with some statistics. According to the CDC from 2020, "46.9 percent of adults aged 18 or older met the Physical Activity Guidelines for aerobic physical activity." (Elgaddal. 2022). This includes running, walking, playing sports, etc. This is in reference to physical activity and suggests that more than 50 percent are not getting enough activity. However, according to the CDC, only "24.2 percent of adults aged 18 and older met the Physical Activity Guidelines for both aerobic and muscle-strengthening activity." (Elgaddal. 2022). This is in reference to those who actively workout and suggests that more than 75 percent of people do not regularly workout.

According to the Annual Review of Public Health from 2005, there has been a decline in physical activity since 1955. In the article "Declining Rates of Physical Activity in the United States: What are the Contributors?" by Ross Brownson, many contributions to this decline in physical activity are discussed. Possibly the largest contributor for the decline in physical activity/exercise is due to a substantial decrease in leisure activities and sports. These leisure activities include cycling, hiking, roller blading, swimming, and even active games like kick the can. A large source of entertainment between the 1950's-1970's was in leisure activities and sports. In 2023, our largest source of entertainment is found in social media, television, and video games.

The rise in media as our source of entertainment is probably the largest reason for a decline in physical activity. What used to be, "Let's meet at the park to play basketball or soccer" is now replaced with "Let's meet online to play basketball and soccer video games." The nature scenes from a bike ride are now being replaced with the scenes from television. Even our social activities of meeting up with friends are being replaced with FaceTime. These are just a few examples of how we are becoming less physically active. **The digital age of**

television and entertainment is keeping us occupied while we sit on the couches of inactivity.

Another large reason for the decline in physical activity that I believe is worth mentioning is the evolution of the workforce. The blue-collar workforce is transitioning into a more white-collar workforce. White-collar jobs generally entail less physical activity than blue-collar jobs. To make inactivity even worse for white-collar workers, between 2019 and 2023, there was a steep increase in remote work amongst mainly white-collar workers due to the pandemic. How much activity can we perform in a house or apartment?

As a blue-collar working personal fitness trainer who uses a step tracker, I will average between 10k-12k steps per day just through performing my job. In fact, when I was a full-time group instructor, I would average between 15k-20k steps per day. Some of my white-collar clients who work remotely have admitted that at the end of the day they've only reached 1.5k-2k steps. Apart from general health, imagine how much of a difference 2k steps per day and 20k steps per day is going to have on someone's physique and cardiovascular health. In fact, when I switched from being a full-time group fitness instructor (15k-20k steps/day), to a full-time personal trainer (10k-12k steps/day), I noticed a pretty dramatic difference in both my physique and cardiovascular health just from a 5k-8k decline in total steps taken per day.

The number one cause of death within the U.S. is cardiovascular disease. Some of my clients that work remotely and don't do cardio outside of our training sessions have fairly severe cardiovascular issues. The number one way to combat and help prevent cardiovascular disease is by doing cardio, exercising, and increasing physical activity. More physical activity and doing cardio has even been beneficial in reducing the risk of Covid fatalities due to its benefits on respiratory health.

Another reason for the decline in physical activity is because of the evolution of lifestyle factors. This includes increased time working especially amongst females in the workforce, increased time in an automobile, an increase in metropolitan population leading to the decrease in environmental space for physical activity, and the increase in apartment living as they require less physical labor to maintain. Our apartments are even being built smaller than ever before. It may seem silly to make this argument, but a remote worker living in a 1200 square foot apartment might be getting twice the activity as a remote worker living in a 500 square foot apartment. Some of us, and I'll admit that I'm referring to myself on this one, rarely go out to go shopping anymore as we buy everything online. A negative side effect of more conveniences is less physical activity.

All these small adjustments in our lifestyle factors are having a negative impact on our activity level and essentially our health and well-being. **It may be hard to admit, but as a society today, we are lazy. The reality is, we are being conditioned to be lazy.** The digital age is promoting laziness with its conveniences. Our workforce is keeping us lazy with shifting workforce expectations. Our small environment with limited in-person social interaction is instilling laziness with the lack of accessibility to activity space. Unfortunately, there is no sign of these trends changing anytime soon, which means we need to be more cognizant of our physical activity than ever before. Many factors have led to an increase in obesity, and I believe that this is one of the chief factors. This is one of our societal roadblocks to success. (Brownson. 2005).

Let's talk about a practical solution to combat inactivity. Inactivity might not be an issue for a large percentage of us, but we all can benefit from more activity. And on the topic of inactivity, I'm definitely speaking to all white-collar remote workers. While the solution may seem as simple as increasing your daily activity, I'm going to give you a tool that is going to help you significantly increase your activity level. Most of my extremely successful clients use this tool, and it's a tool that is an absolute must for my white-collar remote workers. The tool I'm referring to is a fitness tracker. Most come in the form of a watch, such as an Apple Watch, Fitbit, or a Whoop. But some offer chest strap options or even jewelry options such as the Oura. While there are some extremely amazing features on some of the high-end fitness trackers such the Whoop and Oura, any fitness tracker including the $40 knockoffs on Amazon are going to add huge benefit. Some of the most amazing features on even the inexpensive trackers include a step tracker, caloric burn tracker, a heart rate monitor, and a sleep tracker. With some of these fitness trackers, you can even set an activity goal for the day. It will alert you if you are behind on your activity for the day, and it will even give you a notification telling you to stand up and start moving. If your goal is to increase physical activity, the feature that I believe to be the most beneficial is the step tracker. For many of my clients, the step tracker has become a fun daily game and an accountability. It leads to parking the car in the back of the parking lot. It leads to taking the stairs instead of the elevator. It encourages longer walks with the dog.

Wearing a watch with the intended purpose of using it as a fitness tracker always keeps you cognizant of your fitness goals, as it creates a psychological connection and a subtle reminder. Those small shifts in activities will make a huge difference in the physique and overall health. **If you have a goal to burn more calories and improve your cardiovascular health, maybe the solution isn't necessarily to increase your cardio, but to increase your physical activity.** Taking it a step further, make it your goal to increase your intensity in everything you do. Move faster, walk with more intensity, push harder, make yourself more tired. As society pushes for inactivity, it's time to push back with creating a lifestyle built on more activity.

Over-Accessibility

I'm going to tell you something bizarre. The over-accessibility of food is connected to obesity. I'm not about to make a comparison as to why an American is more likely to be overweight than someone from an impoverished country with a lack of food supply. I am going to argue that an environment of over-accessibility can promote overindulgence.

Before I continue, I'm going to remind you of my cruise story from 2022. Do you remember the story of me gaining over 10 pounds in seven days on that cruise? As I've meditated on all the factors that were involved in such a dramatic weight gain, there are two main factors that were apparent. 1. I was constantly hungry, which I believe was largely due to an extreme increase in sugar and carb consumption. 2. I had unlimited access to food as cruise ships have 24/7 buffets. I had an over-accessibility to food, which promoted over-indulgence and weight gain.

So what does this have to do with us?

I recently had an ah-ha moment when I took a trip to visit my friends Pedram and Mel in Austin, Texas. Pedram and Mel are possibly the healthiest couple I've ever met. Apart from the fact that they workout regularly and are very active individuals, they likely have the cleanest and healthiest American kitchen that I've ever been in. I think it is important to know that Pedram is not from the United States. Pedram is Persian, born and raised in Denmark, and has lived in the U.S. for only eight years. In exploring their kitchen, most of what they had in their refrigerator was a small handful of seasonings/dressings in the door, a half dozen healthy energy drinks, a few one gallon water jugs, and a handful of healthy meals that they cook in individual meal prep containers. They have a full-sized refrigerator that was only maybe 30 percent full. In their pantry was only a small handful of healthy snacks like granola bars in the event they ever get extremely hungry and need some fuel, and a few other ingredients for cooking. For the most part, that was it. It's not because they don't have the means to have more food, but in Pedram's words, "We only keep the foods that we need." If your goal is to create a lifestyle of healthy eating, that is the environment of success! That is what your kitchen should look like. Like Pedram, we need to change our mindset about the purpose of food. They don't walk down the grocery aisles asking "What do we want?" They walk down the grocery aisles asking "What do we need?"

While the majority of Americans are fortunate to have the means and accessibility, the environment of over-accessibility within our homes creates the temptations of over-indulgence. If we are honest, most of us have an "American sized refrigerator" that's at least two-thirds full. A large percentage of our homes also have a pantry full of food. Most new builds have walk-in pantries. And then, we have a lot of cabinet space for more food. Many of us probably have enough food to last four weeks without the need to shop for survival. Most of us have the ability in our kitchens to satisfy any craving and every opportunity to feed our feelings! "I feel like eating something sweet… so I will walk downstairs and get something sweet." Some of us might have mostly healthy foods, but even then, you can over-indulge in what's healthy to a point where it becomes unhealthy. Some of us have kitchens that look like a cruise buffet because of the unlimited access to food.

A crop farmer doesn't grow crops, but they create an environment where crops can grow. This is the mindset that we need to have in creating our environment within our home. Some of us are putting ourselves in an environment where it's hard to be successful. Rule number one for an alcoholic going through recovery is don't make alcohol easily accessible by keeping it in the house. Having accessibility will create greater temptation. What if we took on that mentality about food accessibility in our house? What a profound impact that could make! If we want to be successful in our fitness journey, we need to create a healthy environment in our kitchen.

When dialing in on your dieting goals, create an environment for success. This is some of the most simplistic wisdom that I can give you, but some of the most beneficial. Do not keep all those unnecessary foods, especially unhealthy foods, in your house. Take inventory of what you keep around. Truth is, it all starts at the grocery store with what we decide to buy. It requires less discipline to say no to the unhealthy and unnecessary food when you are at the grocery store. It requires more discipline to say no when it's in the pantry and you are sitting on the couch with a late-night food craving. If it's in the pantry, it's overly-accessible. If the craving hits and you have to go to the grocery store to get it, more than likely you won't go through the effort. You are not going to wake up the next day and be mad that you didn't have that late night bag of chips the night prior.

I'm going to let you in on a secret. It's the secret that makes almost all of my personal training clients extremely successful in their fitness and health journey. It's the secret that makes a bodybuilding competitor extremely successful with their physique development. What's the secret? Meal prep.

Meal Prep

Meal prep simply means having meals prepared for the week. This can be done through cooking your own healthy meals or using a meal prep service with pre-cooked meals. Some meal prep services will even send you all the ingredients and recipes for you to cook the meals yourself. I've personally taught myself to fall in love with cooking, so I'll make my own meals. My wife prefers to use a meal prep service with pre-made meals, and she will stack her meals in the refrigerator for each day of the week.

The largest benefit that meal prep has is its ability to help eliminate the desire to feed your feelings. When lunchtime strikes and you only have a 30-minute break, if you don't have a meal already prepped, more than likely you'll revert to an unhealthy fast-food option. After all, it is the option that is typically cheapest and quickest. Most of the fast-food chains market themselves towards the large percentage of individuals who only get the 30-minute lunch break because they provide maximum convenience and quickness. Not having food prepared will lead to us feeding our feelings. "I'm just going to go ahead and get McDonalds today because I'm craving a Big Mac and I need something quick. I can always start watching my diet tomorrow." One unhealthy meal won't destroy progress, but a series of unhealthy meals will. It's not the one meal that creates the unhealthy setback, it's the lack of discipline in preparing the meal. It's easy to get pulled into the unhealthy option if we don't have our meals prepped.

Meal prep is how you control your menu options. A prepared meal gives you one option.

What I find in my experience is if you have a healthy meal prepared for lunch and/or dinner and you know what you are eating, you'll build up your appetite toward your healthy food. Meal prep is one of the most powerful systems that you can create to ensure success in your health and fitness journey.

What if the question went from "Do I want this food?" to "Do I need this food?" It's not about starving yourself and depriving yourself of food intake. It's about fixing the environment that freely gives us the opportunity to feed our feelings. **The moment that you recognize that the benefits of healthy eating outweigh the pleasures of unhealthy eating, then you will be successful.** Don't eat for pleasure, eat for purpose. You will either eat to live, or you will live to eat. And if you eat to live, you'll gain more life! The more snacks you have around, the more temptations to consume unnecessary food. Don't let your house be an environment like a cruise ship where you constantly drink sugary drinks and have unlimited access to food. Prepare what you need. **Promotion demands preparation!** Like Pedram, only keep around what you need. Whether you view food as fuel or whether you view food as a source of pleasure will make a huge difference in your success in your fitness and health journey!

-Chapter 21-
Validation and Manipulation

"We have become the filter generation of unrealistic expectations."
-Trey Patterson

The next two roadblocks are less of a societal roadblock and more of a personal roadblock that is very common within our society. The first roadblock, may not have that strong of an effect on some, but might have a dramatic effect on others. For me, it was the largest roadblock for me developing a sustainable lifestyle change in my health and fitness journey. It's a roadblock that kept me on a viscous and unhealthy cycle of 90 days of dramatic results followed by 90 days of losing those results. In this chapter, I'm going to become vulnerable with you and share a few issues that I faced that were a major hinderance to me reaching even greater success. It wasn't until I was able to completely destroy this roadblock that I was able to obtain my greatest physique and to become the healthiest version of myself. My largest roadblock to success…. The need for validation!

Validation Generation

Thinking back into my younger days, I always wanted to be the class clown. I always wanted to be the center of attention. I always wanted to be seen and heard. And if I wasn't getting the attention that I felt like I wanted and deserved, I would use any means necessary to get that attention. It led to me making several poor choices in schools and even led to school expulsions. The need to have recognition and the need for external validation was deeply rooted within me. Even if you can't relate, we can all relate to how amazing it feels to receive that recognition and validation from others. But if we are not careful, it can become our trap.

Isn't it amazing when you work hard at something, and others notice your hard work? You've been working hard the past two months to lose those 15 pounds, and you post your most recent picture on social media, to get 2-3 people comment on how good you look and the weight you've lost! "Yes, people are noticing!" Everyone wants to be validated as validation makes us feel successful. It's a spike in endorphins. And the lack of validation may make you feel as though you aren't successful. While there is nothing wrong with the validation itself, on the receiving end however, the need for validation can lead to unhealthy behaviors.

I would never have admitted this when I was in my mid-twenties, but my behaviors were easily influenced by the opinions of others. During a competition prep, I would use extremely unhealthy means to build muscle and size. I would jump on a "bulk diet" of eating as many calories, mostly unhealthy calories, to put on as much size as possible. In doing so, I would get multiple compliments daily from those around me. "Wow, you're looking great Trey! I can tell you've been hitting the gym." It's important to add that during this time of competing in bodybuilding and having developed these very unhealthy patterns, I was working in a group fitness gym training an average of 100 clients per day. I felt this need to represent and impress. When I would cycle off of a "bulk diet," I would then cycle on to a "cut diet," a low-calorie healthy diet. When on a "cut diet" I would constantly have people tell me how I look like I had lost a lot of weight. "You've lost a lot of weight especially in your face." I had a handful of people ask me if I was still even working out. And I had a few people even tell me that I looked unhealthy, "Are you feeling okay?" I would not have admitted this in my mid-twenties either but I had always struggled with a pretty severe body dysmorphia, especially during the time when I was doing bodybuilding competitions.

    Body dysmorphia is a psychological illness, and it's the over-obsession of a perceived flaw. There are many forms of body dysmorphia. The most common type of body dysmorphia is when an individual obsesses over not being skinny enough. The individual might be underweight, but when they look at themselves in the mirror, they see themselves as overweight. For me, it was the opposite. I struggled with thoughts of being too skinny and would even view myself as being malnourished when I started losing weight. With my dysmorphia, someone telling me that I've lost a lot of weight was the equivalent of an individual who obsesses about being overweight, being told that they are gaining weight. It was gut-wrenching when I heard those opinions, and it had a huge effect on me because I cared about someone else's opinion of me. I determined my success based on another's opinion of me.

    I began to associate "unhealthy" with results, looking good, and compliments. And I began to associate "healthy" with regress, not looking good, and concerns from others. The compliments for me were simply reinforcing an unhealthy lifestyle. I was getting all this external validation from doing unhealthy things that were internally hurting me. Yet, this external validation made me feel like I was doing something "right." And the negative opinions would pull me back into a never-ending vicious cycle of returning to my unhealthy lifestyle. This need for validation kept me outcome-focused, not process-focused. I wanted to impress people with my physique, I didn't care about the journey to get there. I just wanted to showcase myself on a stage with a trophy in my hand. The need to impress led to dramatic results that would turn to regress. I was stuck on a roller coaster of highs and lows. Dramatic results, loss of results. Surge of confidence, loss of confidence. Feeling good about how I looked, feeling disgusted by what I saw in the mirror. But the worst part was, it kept me trapped in an unhealthy lifestyle that truthfully took years for me to get out of. My progressed dysmorphia even led to me developing a very unhealthy relationship with food. And it was all because I had the need for validation. There were even a few times that someone would tell me that I looked like I had been losing weight, and I was so affected by the comment, that after I got off of work I would pound down 3,000-4,000 calories of fast food out of frustration in a single sitting. To those with a dysmorphia of being overweight, this could be the equivalent of someone communicating to you that you're gaining weight, and you then starve yourself for the rest of the day or even self-induce throwing up. It wasn't until I broke through my need for validation that I was able to create a sustainable long-term lifestyle change.

    I'm going to speak directly to the individual with body dysmorphia and/or to the individual who struggles with the need for validation. The need for validation is a trap and it can become a major catalyst for an unhealthy lifestyle. It can drive us to unhealthy behaviors such as using starvation methods, over/under-eating, using drugs specifically for weight loss purposes, etc. **If you want to create a healthy lifestyle and develop healthy patterns, it's important to realize that someone else's perception of you doesn't matter.** Even in regards to mental health, you will never be fully content and happy with yourself until you shut down others' perceptions of you. Nobody's opinion of you matters. Nobody's comments toward you matters. And truth is nobody's compliments toward you even matters. The reason I say this is because you can't pick and choose what will have an effect over you. If you allow someone's compliments to have an effect on you, you will be giving permission to allow someone's negative opinion of you to have an effect on you. You will only be fully free to succeed to your greatest potential when you can shut down the need for validation in your life. At the end of this chapter, I will further address how to overcome this roadblock to success. But before that, let's address the last major personal roadblock…. The dangers of comparison.

Fake Generation

Scrolling through the Instagram feed… "Wow, that fitness model looks great! What an amazing pic! I want to look like that!"

Most of us probably have a few fitness models that we look up to and even follow on social media, whether they are fitness trainers, bodybuilding or bikini competitors, or just fitness social media influencers. In the fitness network 30 years ago, the status of success as a fitness model was determined by how many, and what magazines or articles the model was featured in. Today, the status of success is determined by how many followers the model can generate. Many of our fitness models gained their initial recognition through bodybuilding or bikini competitions, or through their great success in sports. Some have gained their recognition from their charming and like-able personalities. But nonetheless, every single one of our established fitness models have an impressive physique. Have you ever wondered what goes into the featured photo of the fitness model? While we may assume that a measure of manipulation takes place to capture the impressive physique, many of us are probably not aware of how much manipulation takes place. I want to paint the picture of what is entailed in what you may be comparing yourself to.

I'm going to disclose the fitness modeling secrets and share what goes into capturing the impressive physique, before we had our common filters. Every single fitness model and bodybuilding competitor knows the term "peak week" all too well. Peak week is the week leading up to the competition or photoshoot where there will be extreme manipulation in diet, water intake, sodium intake, etc, to make their physique look its greatest. The goal is to "peak" the body at the exact moment, the exact hour, of the photoshoot or competition. From an aesthetic standpoint, it's very impressive how much fitness models and competitors can manipulate their bodies within that one week. Some can change their physique so dramatically, that in seven days they can become almost unrecognizable. What exactly is entailed in peak week? I'm going to share my protocol on how I peaked my body, which was a huge factor in me placing in some of the hardest NPC men's physique bodybuilding shows in the U.S.

It's seven days out, it's time to peak the body! The first three days I would significantly increase my water intake by drinking about three gallons of water per day. The first two days of my increased water intake, I would also increase my sodium intake by 2-4 times the amount of usual sodium intake. This would make my body retain a lot of water at the beginning of the week, allowing my muscles to fully hydrate. After all, muscle is mainly water. On day three, while still drinking three gallons of water, I would start taking a diuretic and would completely eliminate sodium for the remainder of peak week. Day four, I would consume one gallon of water. Day five, I would consume a 1/2 gallon of water. Day six, I would only consume about three cups of water. And on day seven (competition day), it's no water and only dry food. Many times, I felt like I was going to pass out on day seven due to dehydration.

One thing that I haven't mentioned is that carbohydrate manipulation was vital for making the body peak. For several weeks before peak week and through most of peak week I would be depleted of carbohydrates usually only consuming about 20-30 grams per day. Day five of peak week, I would increase that amount to about 50 grams of very specific complex carbohydrates. Day six, I would increase that amount to 100 grams. And then on day seven, I would consume between 250-350 grams of carbs. This is done to help pull the remaining water in my body back into my muscles giving it fullness and creating a balloon effect within the muscles. Day six was haircut day, full body shave day, smoldering hot epsom salt bath day (which helped eliminate water from under the skin), and spray tan day. On day seven, about one hour before the big moment of being on stage or doing a photo shoot, I would start eating pixie sticks which would help with increasing vascularity by making my veins pop out. In seven days, I will have experienced about a 5-7 pound water weight fluctuation and my body will look extremely different. It's day seven, and my physique is in its "best" condition, yet I'm extremely unhealthy and on the verge of severe dehydration.

I would use this exact tactic for both a competition or a photo shoot. But let's turn the attention to photo shoot day to discuss the "featured photo." On photo shoot day there will be hundreds of different poses, multiple outfits, and 1000+ shots taken in multiple locations and backgrounds, and it's all taken by a professional photographer or even a team of photographers. These photographers are the masters at capturing the best lighting and angles. After looking through 1000+ photo proofs, we'll narrow down all those shots to the top ten best shots, where the angle, pose, and lighting were all in perfect alignment. It's now editing time. The brightness is manipulated, the contrast is manipulated, the sharpness is manipulated amongst many other things making the physique look even better. And those are the 10 pictures, more or less, that get posted on social media. Some of our top fitness models will only do a few photo shoots per year. Yet, with all of the different outfits and locations from the photo shoot, they'll post another picture every week or so. In doing so, it will make them appear as though they look like that 24/7. To give credit where credit is due, our top competitors and models look great without all the adjustments but there is an extreme amount of manipulation that takes place in the physique, photo shoot, and picture editing to give you the picture that you see.

After all secrets shared, this my question to you- Do you really want to compare yourself to or compete with that?

Today, we have software applications and photo filters so complex that you can alter appearance substantially while looking one hundred percent real. We have filters on our phones far more advanced and believable than an experienced editor/photographer could have created 20 years ago. Even artificial intelligence technologies with one click of a button can put a new outfit on the person in the photo and make it look one hundred percent real. There are even apps that you can download that will change your body composition to add fake muscles, make an individual look 20 pounds less, change the facial structure, distort nose size, lip size, etc. And meanwhile, a majority of people simply scrolling through social media wouldn't be able to tell that a single filter was used. Most of us have never seen our favorite fitness influencers and models in person and have nothing to compare the pics to. A large percentage don't look like that or close to that in person, at least not all the time. **Truth is, social media has created a platform where you mainly see people at their best. For many, it's not just their "best," it's their "fake."**

This has created a problem. As a society, we are becoming more fake. And quite frankly, we are being conditioned to accept fake and to become fake.

As a fitness trainer, there have been many times where I've had a client send me a picture of their favorite fitness model, celebrity, or fitness influencer with the desire to have their physique. Most of the time, the pictures are highly manipulated, or they are pictures of individuals who don't have natural physiques due to sports enhancement drugs or steroid use. Fake is becoming more common. Filters are becoming more common. **We have become the filter generation of unrealistic expectations.** You'll never be happy with the outcome if you are chasing after what's unrealistic. Be optimistic, but don't accept unrealistic as it's unattainable.

The first thing that I'd like to say is that we must stop comparing ourselves to others. If not, it will serve as not just a roadblock to success but it will become a roadblock for your own happiness. Comparison is dangerous. In the same way that comparison to other people's "perfect lives" on social media can be a major catalyst for depression, comparison to other people's physiques can be a catalyst for depression in our own physiques. How defeating it will be if you spend years of dieting and countless hours in the gym to find that you are nowhere near to where your role models are at, especially if we aren't aware that we are comparing to what's fake.

Speaking to the individual especially with body dysmorphia, we must be able to separate fake from reality and filters from truth. Filters, photoshop, editing, or whichever term you connect with is a threat to your success. Filters do not portray what is real. A filter won't make you skinny. A filter won't fix blemishes. A filter won't make you healthy. A filter won't give you muscles. In fact, I believe that our filters are the number one reason why more and more are developing body dysmorphia. **A filtered version of you makes the world see a fake version of you, yet makes you see a flawed version of you.** A filter will make you believe you are not skinny enough. A filter will make you believe you look too old. A filter will make you believe that your nose is too big, your cheek bones are too big, your ears are too big, etc. If you are not careful, you'll begin to obsess over a flaw that no one even sees. **You will never produce positive change until you create a positive perception of yourself.** Stop focusing on your flaws and start focusing on your strengths. Only then will you develop a healthy perception to produce healthy change.

For myself, while validation was possibly the largest aggravation to my own body dysmorphia, possibly the largest onset of it was from comparing my current physique to my "photoshoot/filtered" physique. By staring at my filtered photos and even creating an entire social media platform portraying that manipulated image of me, I thought that it would build up my own confidence. But what I was actually doing was feeding a dysmorphia and destroying my own self-esteem as I would wake up in the morning and be disgusted by what I saw, because I didn't look anything like what I was trying to convince myself I did look like. I was actually destroying my confidence. One of the largest contributors to being stuck in an unhealthy lifestyle is because we have an unhealthy image of ourselves. You'll never be free, if you are trying to convince yourself that the fake, manipulated, filtered version of you is the real you. You'll remain in a cycle of not just unhappiness but unhealthiness, if you can't accept the real you. You must break through the fake if you want to be able to grasp who you can really become.

Motivation for You: Love Yourself

We've all heard of the two great commandments. "1. Love the Lord God with all your heart, all your soul, and all your mind. 2. Love your neighbor as yourself." There's something I want to bring to attention with the second command that rarely gets discussed in our churches. Love your neighbor as "yourself." **Self-love is the most important physical relationship goal that you should ever have.**

You will only manifest to the world what you are nurturing internally. And you will only manifest to yourself what you are nurturing internally.

The most effective change is rooted in self-love. If you spend your time tearing yourself down with the mindset that self-hatred will actually produce change, it will never produce a healthy lifestyle change. If you are someone who struggles to love yourself or you are someone with severe body dysmorphia, my greatest advice to you would be to take time every day, look at yourself in the mirror and point out your attractive features. It doesn't just have to be a physical feature, it could be a strength that you possess. I do have beautiful eyes.

My arms do look good. I am a strong leader at my job. I am a strong performer at work. I am a good mother. I guarantee you that if you take the time to search for your attractive features or your strengths, you will find them. When your attractive features and your strengths become the point of recognition, it will destroy your obsession over your perceived flaws. It will destroy your dysmorphia. And more than anything it will lead to a greater self-love.

Truth is, we are being conditioned at a social level not to love ourselves. And it's leading to a rising industry of people profiting off of your insecurity. We have filters altering our appearance to make us look more "beautiful," "younger," "skinnier," etc. Then every time we look in the mirror we see our "flaws." Meanwhile, people see a filtered/photoshop version of us on social media and compliment us on how good we look. Many of us get trapped by the need for validation, and it leads to an unhealthy version of us or a need to create an even greater filtered/photoshop version of us. Don't compare yourself to others' looks and lives on social media. You're not seeing behind the curtain. You're not seeing behind the filter. You're not seeing truth. You're only seeing what they want you to see.

When you develop self-love, no one else's opinions of you will matter. When your actions aren't influenced by others' opinions of you, only then will you walk in freedom. Self-love is freedom!

You'll never have shame in yourself if you love yourself. Self-love isn't about trying to be someone else, it's about being the best version of yourself. Self-love will compel you to be a healthier, stronger, and a better version of you. Self-hatred pushes you into an unhealthy lifestyle while self-love promotes a healthy lifestyle. If you are trapped in disappointment, if you're trapped in self-hatred, if all you see is your flaws, I'm going to give you an assignment. Take 30 seconds every single day and listen to yourself breathe. That's evidence that you have life. While you're upset about your flaws and your weaknesses, while you are disappointed, while you have self-hatred, someone no longer even has that opportunity to take another breath. When you take those 30 seconds every day to listen to yourself breathe, meditate on how lucky you are to be alive.

You can't put a price tag on yourself because you are worth everything! Even to someone else, you are worth everything. Almost everyone that has recently passed away currently has someone on this earth that would give up everything they own to have them back on this earth. There is not a greater God-given asset than your own body and your own life, so love yourself enough to make yourself a priority. If you love yourself enough, it will have a positive effect on every area of your life. It will increase your desire to make healthy choices. It will increase your desire to exercise. It will increase your desire to eat healthy. In doing so, your day-to-day functions will become easier. Your attitude will become better. Your confidence will increase. And your self-perception will improve. Factually speaking, you will even prolong your life. Loving yourself will produce not just more life, but a greater quality of life. Money can't buy health, or buy back the years of neglected health. Give your family and children a one hundred percent healthy version of you, as you are worth more than any financial investment to them. We've got one life to live. So love yourself and feed yourself with more life.

-Chapter 22-
Small Steps, Distance Traveled

"It's a series of small steps that seem so insignificant at the time that you are making them. Then you look back and realize the distance traveled."
-Tom Brady

Goals are an essential part of life and success. All of us have goals, whether they are conscious or subconscious goals. When we think of goals, we naturally think of our conscious goals such as "I want to see my abs by summer," or "I want to make a six-figure income by the age of 30." However, goals subconsciously come into your mind every day without you even realizing it. A subconscious goal can be "I have to leave the house and head to work at 8 a.m." with the goal of arriving by 8:30 a.m. If you have physique goals, every time that you think about eating, physique goals subconsciously come to your mind and may shift your actions and behaviors.

Without goals, we would wander aimlessly. Without goals, there is no growth as goals provide the opportunity for growth. There's no limit to how many goals you should create, as long as you are willing to commit to accomplishing those goals. The creation of goals subconsciously changes your thought process, gives clear direction, and compels new actions. For example, knowing that you have an established goal of eliminating unhealthy snacks will change how you respond when walking down the grocery aisle where they keep the unhealthy snacks.

Over the next three chapters, I want to help you create goals, keep on course in the pursuit of your goals, and help you successfully hit your goals. We need a variety of long-term goals and short-term goals.

Long-term goals are important as they allow you to aim for a greater future or higher purpose. You can have a long-term goal of becoming a marathon runner. You can have a long-term goal of being a home buyer. You can have a long-term goal of becoming a writer. You can have a long-term goal of being an entrepreneur. You can have long-term goal of one day becoming a millionaire. Every single one of these examples that I give of long-term goals are identity-based. Again, the outcome of the highest achievement is in the development of a new identity. **We may certainly have a long-term goal of accomplishing something, but if you want to see a sustainable change, the goal shouldn't just be about accomplishing something, it should be about becoming something or someone.**

Before any short-term goal is created, you must have established your long-term goals. In terms of duration, I would refer to a long-term goal as any goal that has a duration of two years or more. "I want to become a triathlete in two years. I want to become a business owner in five years. I want to be an entrepreneur and own several businesses in ten years. I want to be retired in twenty years." Long-term goals are central to all of our dreams and aspirations. While many of our long-term goals will change, establishing these goals will guide us in a progressive direction. In fact, without long-term goals, it will be difficult to develop short-term goals. While long-term goals are important, I believe short-term goals are the lifeline of accomplishing those long-term goals. Short-term goals are the goals that we can pursue here and now.

Let's lean in on the topic of short-term goals. Within this chapter, I'm going to help you establish what a short-term goal is. Over the next couple chapters, I'm going to help you create goals and help you create a strategy to conquer those goal.

In terms of duration, I would define a short-term goal as a goal that you'd like to accomplish within three months. In bodybuilding competition, the preparation time for a competitor varies from person to person, but a very standard prep time is about three months (12 weeks). Why? You can have a very dramatic change in your physique within three months. Three months is also a near term goal that will be easier to focus on compared to a 2-5 year goal. It's a goal within your current grasp. This duration of time has been proven to be effective for competition prep. And because three months is within closer grasp, it will also be easier to keep your motivation, discipline, and optimism high. A key component of many short-term goals is to create new habits.

Three months is an effective duration of time for a short-term goal because it's also in alignment with what's called the 21/90 rule. If you're not familiar with the 21/90 rule, it was developed by Dr. Maxwell Maltz, who made the claim that it takes 21 days to form a new habit, and 90 days (3 months) to break an old habit. New habits being formed, and old habits being broken, are what lead to a new outcome and the creation of a lifestyle change.

I want you to visualize a tree. Think of long-term goals as the tree and short-term goals as the roots. Without the roots, the tree won't grow or develop. When you water a tree, you're not going to focus on spraying the water on the branches and leaves. You're going to focus on spraying water on the soil around the tree to nourish the roots of the tree. If you focus on the short-term goals, your long-term goals will naturally come to fruition. If you want to grow into your destiny, if you want to grow into your purpose, if you want to accomplish your long-term goals, focus on the short-term goals. In fact, you may far exceed your long-term goals through repeated success in your short-term goals.

Success in the evolution of your long-term goals comes from the nourishment of your short-term goals. Once you accomplish your short-term goals, create new short-term goals. If you are struggling with a goal, create a new goal. But most importantly, don't grow complacent with your goals. Because short-term goals should only last a few months, you should constantly be creating new short-term goals. Short-term goals are just stepping stones. They should be easy to reach and they shouldn't take long to reach. If long-term goals are the finish line, the short-term goals are your milestones.

Recently, I was watching a documentary on Tom Brady on ESPN+ called "Man in the Arena." It's a documentary on the life and career of Tom Brady where they interviewed several of Tom Brady's teammates, previous coaches, family members, and of course, several interviews with Tom Brady himself. In one of the interviews, he was asked what he believed led to his great success. This interview took place after Tom Brady won his 7th Super Bowl while playing for the Buccaneers. This is the statement he made about his success - "It's a series of small steps that seem so insignificant at the time that you are making them. Then you look back and realize the distance traveled."

The short-term goals are the small steps, and distance traveled is the recognized accomplishment of your long-term goals. Create short-term goals based upon areas where you want to see small improvements, as the short-term goals should pave the way for those small improvements. A series of small improvements lead to a big improvement over time. When you keep making those small improvements, this is the essence of transformation and a major part of the process of change and transformation.

Motivation for You: There's Power in Small

There is power in taking small steps forward. Embrace the small steps or those small, short-term goals. The only danger that you have is when you are no longer moving forward and taking those steps. Because life moves forward, if you are at a standstill then you are actually digressing. If you stop in a race, you don't remain in your position, you'll get further behind. It's because we live in a competitive world. A lot of what you may think are insignificant steps will one day lead to a significant difference. You may be in a place where you feel like you've been taking small steps and you haven't seen change. You've been working and training hard, yet you have not seen much benefit. That's nothing but the challenge of your endurance. Challenge is what makes you stronger.

Metaphorically speaking, how many marathons could you finish if you just keep taking those small steps? How many mountains could you climb if you just keep taking the small steps? How many great things can you accomplish if you just keep moving forward? No glory goes to a person who runs 3/4 of a marathon at a great speed then quits. The person who finishes, even if it takes them longer, still gets a reward. It's better to be late, than never show up. It's better to take longer, than never finish.

There will be a lie that will try and creep into your head. "My glory days are behind me." "I'm too old." "I'm too young." "That's not realistic for me to accomplish something that big." Those thoughts are the great lie. Biologically, your entire existence from fetus, to baby, to a grown adult was a miraculous process. This is evidence that you were born to do miraculous things. The human mind has yet to align with our human capability as our potential is endless.

Don't be afraid to take your first steps. Sometimes we see these wildly successful people and think to ourselves, "There's no way I can do that." Jeff Bezos started Amazon with nothing more than an idea in his head and more than likely, he had no idea how wildly successful his business would become and how one day he would dominate e-commerce. He probably did not have a game plan in place to support a billion-dollar business prior to creating Amazon. It all started with one step forward. It started with the goal to start a business. Like any major business, Jeff Bezos faced many roadblocks, had financial concerns, and hit learning curves that forced him to become more educated in certain legalities. There are some things that you will only learn through experience. You'll never know what can trip you if you are never taking steps. This is life! Jeff Bezos one day became the richest man in the world and one of the most successful men of all time. It was because he kept taking step after step.

How does this relate to you? Despite every tough time you've gone through in your life, every financial battle you've ever had, any curve ball that you've ever had to deal with, you survived! Not only have you survived, but your experience led to new knowledge. A lot of the knowledge we have gained in life were lessons learned through unfortunate circumstances. There will be times when you hit roadblocks. There will be times when you hit learning curves. There will be times when you fight plateaus. This is all a vital part of the process. But you will never be successful if you never take the first step. You don't have to figure everything out before you start, just start by creating movement. In the same fashion that you've figured out everything that life has thrown your way, you will figure out how to become successful.

Even after all those times that you make the decision to go workout, or all those times that you decide to go with the healthier food option, you may not see a difference after your first 1, 2, even 10 times. One day you will see the difference as long as you keep putting one foot in front of the other. It is important to add that this also works the opposite way, I'll refer to these steps backward as setbacks. A setback occurs with two steps. We rationalize, then we compromise. You won't notice a difference with one unhealthy meal, but you'll notice a difference when that unhealthy meal leads to a habit of eating unhealthy meals. It doesn't matter how strong you are, almost every single one of us will have setbacks. The great test is that you keep making the effort to take steps forward even when you feel defeated. This is the reason why short-term goals are powerful. They will draw you back into taking positive actions and draw you back into healthy habit formations.

Tests are inevitable. **Like any school test you've ever taken, tests are less about demonstrating your knowledge, and they are more about bringing an awareness to what we don't know.** The test will show us our opportunity for growth. Unlike a school test, the only way we fail our tests in life is if we quit. Turn your test into a testimony. Growth mentality creates the ability to learn from mistakes and creates the ability to turn a setback into a comeback. You didn't come this far, just to make it here. You got to where you are because you didn't give up. Today is just your stepping stone to an even better path. Everyday is the first day of a greater day. Your better days lie ahead of you. There will be some days where it may not feel like it's your best day, but as long as you don't quit, one day you'll look back and notice the upward trend.

The only wall, the only true barrier that will stop you from fully living out your dreams, is when you say, "I can't." Just because someone else failed, doesn't mean you will too. **Don't let someone else's success, or lack of success, be your standard. You are your own author, so pick up your pen and write.** Small steps lead to distance traveled.

-Chapter 23-

Make Creative Goals

"The aggressive approach that leads to a burnout may yield quick results, but it will also keep you trapped in the roller coaster of highs and lows."
-Trey Patterson

There is probably not a topic that more books have been written about than goal creation. In the previous chapter, we discussed the importance of short-term goals and how the short-term goals are those small steps toward your greater goals. Within this chapter, I'm going to give you practical insight on how to successfully create those short-term goals.

If you are someone that really struggles accomplishing your goals, someone that has a tendency to quickly give up on your goals, or someone that no longer likes to even set goals because you've been unsuccessful in hitting all your previous goals, I would attribute that lack of success to four things. 1. You have uncreative/non-exciting goals. 2. You haven't done a self-assessment to create realistic goals. 3. You lack the motivation to reach for those goals. 4. You have an ineffective action plan. These are four topics that I'll be discussing over the next couple of chapters. While my discussion of goals can be utilized for goals outside of fitness goals, I'm going to specifically speak to fitness goals.

Before we start creating our goals and address the reasons why we maybe haven't successfully reached our previous goals, let's talk about the big fitness goal. It's the goal that probably a majority of people reading this have. It's usually the reason why we start our exercise and dieting regimen... Weight loss! Weight loss is a term that I've used frequently in this book because it's the term we are accustomed to.

Let us actually break apart the idea of weight loss. As a society, we've become too attached to the term "weight loss." Weight is a measurement determined by a scale. "Loss" implies a decrease in the measurement determined by the scale. **I'm going to make a bold statement: general weight loss should never be a fitness goal.** There are a lot of different kinds of weight that you can lose. You can lose muscle weight. Quick reminder, muscle weighs more than fat. You can lose fat weight. You can lose water weight. You can even lose bone density weight. I repeat, weight loss should never be a fitness goal. For those with the weight loss goal, the goal should truly be "body fat reduction." With the body fat reduction goal, weight loss is almost bound to occur, but the focus should never be a number on a scale.

I'm not an advocate for weight goals for most of my clients and for many reasons. I've even pulled away from using a scale with most of my clients, unless it's to track body fat percentage. Many of my clients will obsess about that weight number as if it's their badge of accomplishment. And in a lot of cases, many of my clients will even revert to an unhealthy means to reach a certain number, just so they can feel accomplished. Now, I will say that using a scale may be different for everyone as many don't have an unhealthy relationship with the scale. If I recognize that a client may have body dysmorphia or an eating disorder, I will never use a scale. In fact, if you struggle with an eating disorder or body dysmorphia, do not keep a scale around the house. There are healthier ways to track progress and for those with body dysmorphia or an eating disorder, it will only intensify a dysmorphia or an eating disorder. If you are someone who falls into this category and perceive you have an unhealthy obsession with a weight goal yet still want to track progress, I would highly recommend using a hand-held body fat reader such as the Omron body fat percentage reader. In fact, when I competed in bodybuilding competitions, it's the only scale I used because a regular scale would be a distraction from my goal of decreasing body fat percentage.

    Another detrimental feature that I find about the general weight loss goal is that weight is easily manipulated. I've had multiple previous clients admit to me before a weigh-in that they haven't had anything to eat or drink all day so that they could have a better weigh-in. On the flip side, I can drink a high calorie protein shake, drink two bottles of water, then jump on the scale to find out I'm four pounds heavier than 30 minutes prior. Everyone fluctuates between 2-4 pounds per day in water weight. If you weigh yourself in the morning you will probably weigh at least 2-3 pounds less than when you weigh yourself in the evening because the body dehydrates during sleep. After a month, a basic weight loss number could show that you are down three pounds, but your body fat may have increased by two percent. This means that the weight you've lost was almost all muscle weight or water weight. When I competed in bodybuilding competitions, I could easily lose over five pounds within 24 hours before my show by taking a diuretic, smoldering epsom salt bath, dehydration, and the elimination of sodium. It was all water weight. My point is that the general weight goal isn't really an accurate measurement. For many, it's easy to develop an unhealthy relationship with a scale.

Creative Goals

Let's turn the topic back to how to create goals. As mentioned earlier, I would attribute the lack of success to four things, with one of them being we have uncreative goals. So what are "uncreative goals?" Creating goals requires creativity. Let me give you an example of an uncreative goal versus a creative goal. "I want to lose 30 pounds within 3 months" versus "I want to drop 2-3 dress sizes within three months." The latter is a more creative goal, and I believe a far more effective "weight loss" goal. For a guy, a creative goal could be, "I want to fit into that collared shirt that I wore two years ago at the Christmas party." I personally have used this tactic through my years of competing in bodybuilding. I would make it my goal to grow into my larger shirts during bulk time. For me, it served as a huge motivation tactic, and it would generate much more motivation than hitting a weight number. Nothing excited me more during my prep than growing into my larger shirts, and I would wear that larger shirt as a badge of accomplishment. For a female, it could be fitting into that dress. How exciting would it be to fit into that dress you loved but haven't been able to wear in three years? A creative goal like this is tangible, further enhancing motivation, discipline, confidence, and the desire to continue. Being motivated and developing discipline in the pursuit of your goals are the two key ingredients to being successful at hitting your goals.

Part of developing creative goals is developing a diversity of goals. If your only goal is to look better aesthetically, there will be days, even entire seasons, when you may not be content with how you look. That's a motivation crusher. There will even be times when you are content with how you look. While that's great, we should always strive for improvement. Have strength goals like bench pressing a certain weight. Have fitting into your favorite pants goals. Have body fat percentage goals.

If your goals don't excite you, it will be hard to keep the motivation and discipline to pursue your goals. I can tell you with almost one hundred percent certainty that you will not be successful in hitting your goals if you have a negative attitude about your goals. Creating goals that excite you will allow you to stay focused on the process. I've never seen someone completely transform their physique while rolling their eyes through the entire process. I believe that this is part of the reason why many may struggle with their New Year's resolution fitness goals. Every year it has become an un-exciting ritual of "It's January 1st, I have to start dieting and exercising again." I'm by no means bashing a New Year's resolution, as I think setting goals at the beginning of a new year is a great time to set goals. But I'm specifically commenting on how for many, the New Year's resolution has become a forced action that isn't exciting. For many, the resolution was created out of shame from the poor lifestyle habits created during the holidays. Excitement in your goals keeps you on the pursuit of your goals. And the purpose of creating goals is to keep you on the pursuit of self-improvement.

The Power of Self-Assessment

Creating goals also requires self-assessment. While there are many questions that you can ask to assess yourself, I'm going to list the five most important questions. And I highly encourage you to take the time to reflect on these questions. It's only through self-assessment that you can effectively create the right goals for you. My purpose as a coach is to help you come to self-realization, actualization, and help you discover the greater you. A self-assessment to better understand yourself is an important aspect in creating realistic goals and it will allow you to clearly see how aggressive your goals should be.

1. What is my current availability to pursue my goals? This one is pretty self-explanatory. Your availability can paint the picture of how much time you are able to commit to those goals.

2. What is my current emotional state/well-being? What is my stress level? If you are in a fragile emotional state or have high levels of stress, then you may not want to create extremely aggressive goals. On the flip, if you are in a strong emotional state with low levels of stress, the creation of more aggressive goals may be a better alignment.

3. Am I naturally a more optimistic or pessimistic individual? Whether you are naturally more optimistic or pessimistic won't just influence the kind of goals you create, it will influence the actions you implement in the pursuit of those goals.

4. What was my success rate with my previous goals? If there was a lack of success, discover what the variables were that interfered with that lack of success.

5. What is my motivation level? This is the self-assessment that I'm about to focus on and break down in detail.

If you are reading this book, there is a high probability that you are highly motivated. As a personal trainer, one of the first things I'll seek to recognize in an onboarding client is their motivation level. If they communicate to me that they are not very motivated, I will never recommend them working out five times per week, no matter how aggressive their initial goals might be. That would not be a realistic goal. I've eavesdropped on many trainers in the gym and have listened to them try and push all of their clients to work out everyday. "Let's do this again tomorrow. And the next day. You said you want to get results right?"

If you are just starting on your fitness journey, new habits will not form overnight. And if you're not motivated in the pursuit of your goals, a burnout is almost bound to happen if you are too aggressive with your goals. When a burnout occurs, it's hard to re-ignite the flame. **The aggressive approach that leads to a burnout may yield quick results, but it will also keep you trapped in the roller coaster of highs and lows.** A burnout will create an unsustainable pattern, and it's a threat to the process of transformation.

If you feel strong and confident after your self-assessment about your ability to reach your goals, you may have the ability to be more aggressive with your goals. Be aggressive, but not unrealistic. There is a fine line between aggressive goals and unrealistic goals. Unrealistic goals do not pave the way to success. Should you expand your vision and shoot for the stars? Absolutely! I definitely want you to be optimistic as well. It's through your self-assessment that you better understand what goals are right for you and what you are capable of accomplishing. The accomplishment of a realistic goal should produce optimism. Again, don't brush off those small goals as being insignificant. You'll become far more optimistic by accomplishing three small goals than you will by struggling to accomplish that one big goal.

If you are setting fitness goals and you lack motivation, that's understandable. At least you're setting goals, and you're one step ahead of most. If your motivation is low, your biggest fitness goal should be to find more motivation. As I mentioned previously, I'm going to share very practical insight in this chapter, and I'm going to share with you my favorite tactics for stimulating my motivation levels.

Get Motivated

One of my biggest pet peeves is when I hear motivational speakers talk about why motivation is not important. A little ironic, isn't it? Many books have been written on the topic of why motivation isn't important, and why discipline is what you actually need in order to succeed. As if it's a choice that you can only have one or the other. In fact, there have been more books written on why motivation is not important than why it is important. **There are many components needed to produce success, and they all have their function and importance.**

Whether you are currently motivated or not, there is always room to increase your motivation levels. You have to continuously search within yourself and ask the question- Am I really motivated and excited about my goals or am I just going through the motions? If you are just going through the motions, it will be extremely hard to follow a long-term plan. The reality is, motivation will waver. But it's important to always put yourself in an environment of inspiration and motivation. In addition to the simplistic measures such as placing yourself in the right environment and discovering what you enjoy, I'm going to give you my four personal practical ideas that you can draw on for motivation on a daily basis.

1. Write down upcoming important dates when you want to showcase success- weddings, family gatherings, beach vacations, photo shoots, etc. Booking a photo shoot or a vacation creates a specific time frame. If I'm spending money on a photo shoot, it will give me that extra push. And who doesn't want to look their best on vacations especially knowing that the camera is going to be hot.

2. Watch fitness or health videos. YouTube is a great place for this. Whether your goal is losing weight or bodybuilding, you will find a video that inspires you to exercise. Putting that positivity on your screen will enhance optimism that will keep you motivated. Some of these motivational videos come in the form of a fitness/health related docu-series for education, which leads me to my next practical idea.

3. Submerse yourself in education. Read articles about fitness, different exercise concepts, health articles, and of course, books. Not a reader? Listen to those podcasts and audiobooks. When you submerse yourself in fitness education, you will be eager to apply what you've learned to your fitness regimen. Knowledge also increases your confidence, and you'll have

more motivation if you are confident. You may not have been successful before, but maybe in your quest for knowledge comes a solution that will lead to your future success. Knowledge is power. Some of the most successful people are simply the product of what they know.

4. Discover your "why." I believe that this is possibly the strongest motivation tactic. There is a why within all of us, and in the last chapter, I'm going to help you discover it.

-Chapter 24-
It's Action Time

"Goals are stepping stones to an even greater and ever-changing goal."
-Trey Patterson

There are many great books, articles, and courses that have very differing views on what goals are, how to create goals, how to implement goals, etc. Truthfully, I don't think there is anything that I've ever read about goals that didn't bring value. My insight on what I believe are the most effective goals, are in alignment with S.M.A.R.T. goals. If you aren't familiar with S.M.A.R.T. goals, it's an abbreviation for Specific, Measurable, Achievable, Realistic, and Timely. Before we discuss the implementation of those goals, I'd like to add one last point to help you with the creation of goals. Be specific and timely.

Be specific with your goals. Don't be vague. If you have a short-term goal of dropping two dress sizes, instead of creating the goal "I want to drop two dress sizes over the next few months," create a specific timetable. "I want to drop two dress sizes by August 15, two days before my daughter's wedding." When it comes to goals, set dates and be specific. "One day" will never come. To take it a step further, don't just make it your goal to exercise three times per week. Be specific and schedule it into your calendar. "I will exercise on Mondays, Wednesdays, and Fridays at 5:30 p.m." It has been proven that the more specific you are with your goals, the more likely you are to carry out the actions to accomplish those goals. Think of being specific with goals like a dart board. If your goal is to throw that dart as close as you can to the center of the target, you are going to focus on the one-inch red circle in the middle of that board. That one-inch red circle is the specific goal. If you don't have a specific target, you'll be throwing a dart at the large target, and the outcome won't be nearly as precise in comparison to aiming at that specific target point.

Being specific also helps with habit formation and developing routines. You can create a habit of exercising Monday, Wednesday, and Friday at 5:30 p.m. If you are serious about your goals, you'll set it in your calendar and make it a priority.

Action Time

Now that we've discussed goals, I'm going to illustrate to you what I believe to be the most successful way to implement goals. Many of the books, articles, and courses on goals mention creating goals as well as sub-goals. I'm going to use this same illustration but change the verbiage. Instead of sub-goals, I'm going to refer to them as action plans.

There are some people who are highly motivated and create awesome goals, but the reason they don't succeed is because of the lack of an action plan or an ineffective action plan. The plan is just as important as the goal itself, if not more important, as the plan sets the framework for application. Just like the goal requires a creative effort, the plan requires a creative effort as well.

For some, an action plan has a negative stigma. If an employee is underperforming at their job, the boss will put them on an action plan, or sometimes referred to as a PIP (performance improvement plan), which consists of a list of actions with the goal of increasing performance. If you've ever been on a performance improvement plan or action plan with your job, it's neither glorious nor exciting. However, that's an action plan that someone created for you so let's remove the negative connotation. An action plan that you create for yourself should be exciting. If you have already created goals for yourself, this is proof that you have a growth mindset and you desire improvement. The action plan leads to the improvement of your personal performance.

A clear action plan keeps you on course in the pursuit of your goals, which is crucial in accomplishing your goals. Metaphorically speaking, let's discuss building a house. If you want to be successful in building a house, you'll create a blueprint. You'll get the needed tools and machines. You'll hire the labor, and then you'll start to prepare the foundation. These are your plans. The goal is to build the house and the plans pave the way to success. Can you imagine how long it would take to accomplish the task of building a house without a floor plan? Sometimes you'll make mistakes, fix them, then keep building. But, if you just keep working on the plan, you'll eventually succeed and get the outcome that you were looking for. A goal without a plan is simply a dream.

An action plan does require a measure of motivation as it involves implementation. Everything is easier said than done. The question may come to mind, "How many plans should I create for a single goal?" This question takes us back to the idea of self-assessment. To give practical advice, I would suggest that if you aren't very motivated, begin with one or two action plans per goal. If you are highly motivated, create three or four action plans. Self-assessment is not just important with creating goals, but it is just as important to use self-assessment when creating an action plan.

To give practical insight, let's say that you aren't very motivated but you have a goal to increase your motivation levels. Take that goal, and now write down two plans to accomplish that goal. Think of creating plans as creating the blueprint for success. Two action plans for this goal can be "1. I'm going to dedicate 20 minutes per day to reading health and fitness articles. 2. I'm going to listen to a David Goggins audiobook on my drive to work Mondays, Wednesdays, and Fridays." Or let's say that you have a goal of dropping eight percent body fat over the next three months and you assess that you are highly motivated. Three action plans can look like this: "1. I'm going to take a spin class every Monday and Friday at 5:15 p.m., and a group HIIT class every Wednesday and Saturday at 6:30 a.m. 2. I'm going to meal prep every Monday at 7 p.m. and cook 12 healthy meals for the week. 3. I'm going to track my steps on my Apple Watch and hit 12,000 steps every day." If you currently don't workout at all, even if you are highly motivated, two spin classes and two HIIT classes per week may be too aggressive of an action plan. Maybe start off with two total classes per week. If you don't enjoy cooking don't put it in your plans to cook 12 healthy meals each week. Instead, try a meal prep service and replace one meal per day with the meal prep. This illustration is just an example, and an action plan to success is never one-size-fits-all. The plans should fit your personality.

If you are highly motivated, you can create as many action plans as you'd like as long as you know you'll stay committed to the pursuit of those plans. **But sometimes more is not always better. The greater**

goal is to take small steps forward to effectively form new habits. You will not completely transform yourself overnight as the creation of new outcomes is a long process. Your plan is your blueprint to successfully hit your goals, and just like creating goals, the plans should be realistic, easy to follow, a creative reflection of your personality, and enjoyable. On a side note, I'm a big advocate for writing your goals and action plans and putting them in clear sight. In fact, for many of my clients, I'll recommend that they write down their goals on a sticky note and post them on their bathroom mirror. It will be one of the first things that will be noticed every morning upon waking up. Visibility will allow you to see clearly and will build reinforcement.

Creating goals and an action plan requires constant evaluation. Just like in business, you need to evaluate which action plans are creating success, and which ones aren't. Draw more attention to the plans that are producing and cut out the ones that aren't. It's important to re-assess yourself and your action plans at least once a month. Just like most businesses create a KPI (Key Performance Indicator) report on a monthly basis, create a KPI on your action plans. Just as your short-term goals to accomplish your long-term goals are ever-changing, your action plans to accomplish your short-term goals should be ever-changing. No business will ever be successful without creating clear plans for the path to success. It's promotion time; its time to become the COO (Chief Operating Officer) of your own fitness journey.

If long-term goals are like a tree and short-term goals are the roots of the tree, then the action plan is the fertilizer, soil, and water for the roots. The right fertilizer, soil, and water will lead to the nourishment of the roots (short-term goals). Through the nourishment of the roots, the tree (long-term goals) develops. Your tree will only grow to the extent of your nourishment and effort.

(Diagram- Goals)

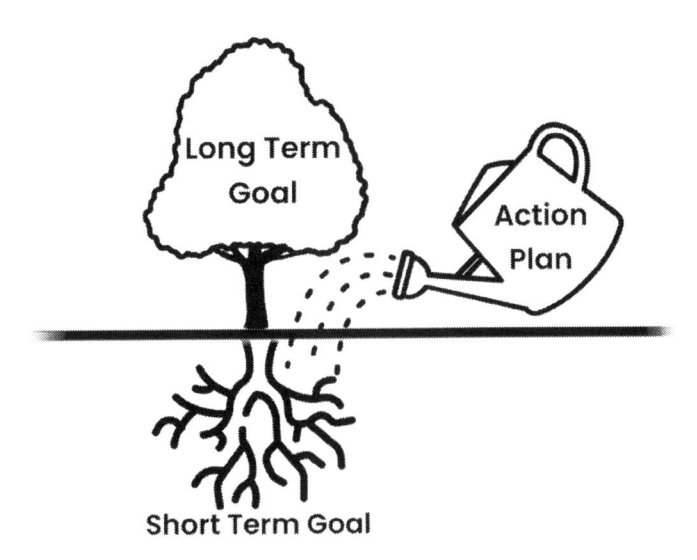

Long Term Goal

Action Plan

Short Term Goal

That last thing I'd like to leave you with on the topic of goals is that goals are not the finish line. **Goals are stepping stones to an even greater and ever-changing goal.** The essence of transformation is a sustained lifestyle that's ever changing. Transformation cannot happen without a goal, so always create new goals to create new change. Don't ever become complacent in your position.

Discover the creative person that you are. Create goals that excite you. Assess yourself and ask yourself the questions before creating those goals. Be optimistic but don't be unrealistic. Be time specific. And last, fight to find the motivation within you.

-Chapter 25-
The Life of Purpose

"Discovering your why is the glue that keeps you connected to your goals."
-Trey Patterson

I can't remember the last time I watched anyone accomplish something great without having at least a small measure of motivation. Motivation is the gunpowder behind firing the gun. It's what is going to give you your rapid push. Without any gunpowder, don't expect to travel far. Don't expect to reach your target. What good are goals and action plans if you are not even motivated to accomplish them? If you are not motivated with the fitness goals or plans you've created, you probably will not last long in your fitness regimen.

In Chapter 23, I gave you my four favorite tactics to enhance motivation. As mentioned, I'm going to expand on the fourth tactic. You must discover your "why."

Discovering your why is the glue that keeps you connected to your goals. Do you remember when you were motivated enough to start your transformation journey? Where did that motivation come from? It started with a "why." More than likely, your why had a subconscious influence that caused you to start a new journey and create your goals. It is important to identify that why. What led to that motivation to change?

It's time to do another self-assessment and it's time to do some soul-searching. I want you to write down your three biggest reasons why you've started your transformation journey or why you've created your goals. This requires meditation. For example... I want to build confidence. To look better. To impress someone. To perform better. To be healthier. To be happier. To be sickness-free.

_____
_____
_____

There is Power in Your Why

Every time that you feel like quitting on your goals, you need to remember your why. Remembering your why is simply keeping the gasoline in hand that sparked the initial fire. It will keep the flame burning. Your why can even be that daily reminder. It can even be that reminder when you feel that tiredness from a run or that pain from a repetition. "I'm willing to embrace the tiredness and willing to embrace the pain because I have a why."

It's time to put a little spin on your why. Now that you've written down your why, I want you to review it. If every why is about you, I want you to add at least two more "whys" that have nothing to do with you. For example... I want to be an example to my kids. I want to inspire my husband/wife to exercise as well. I want to give the best health to those around me. My husband/wife wants me to be healthy.

God wants me to be healthy. I want to set an example for my best friend. I want to pass good health to future generations.

_____

_____

Having a why that revolves around you is the glue that keeps you connected to your goals, and it will give you a reason to pursue your goals. But if you can create a why that is bigger than you, it will strengthen that bond. **The more selfless the why is, the stronger the bond is between you and your goals.**

If your why is selfish and stops at you, your motivation will discontinue when the road gets tough for you. If your why stops at you, you will quit the moment that you believe you achieved it. What's going to happen when you obtain that personal gain? What's going to happen when self-contentment sets in? It's totally fine to be content, but, if you want to reach the higher heights, if you want to go to deeper depths, if you want to go the greater lengths, if you want to experience the greater successes, if you want to have a greater bond and commitment to your goals, you have to find a why that is bigger than you!

When your why becomes selfless, this is the realization that will take place. Your success doesn't just affect you but extends to those beyond you. The decisions you make will affect more than just you. Whether you know it or not, you have an audience that's watching you. You have someone looking up to you. You have someone who is influenced by you. Your kids are watching you. Your family members are watching you. Your friends are watching you. Your followers on social media are watching you. To take it beyond your audience, you have future generations relying on you. Even if you only have an audience of one, that is one person who is affected by your choices. **Everyone is a leader because everyone leads someone.**

Let me tell you what I'm really talking about in terms of discovering a why that is bigger than you. If you can create goals, if you can discover your why, and if you can create a why that is bigger than you, you will discover your purpose. In fact, the discovery of your purpose is a formula. Goals + Why + Selfless Why = Purpose. The reason that so many people are unsuccessful in reaching their goals is because there is a lack of purpose.

There's Power in Purpose

Now when I use the word purpose, it's a word that can mean something different to different people. For some, it's a word about intention. For some, it's of a faith and spiritual nature. For some, it's a word linked to fulfillment and meaning. A psychologist from the University of California Berkeley defined purpose as "an abiding intention to achieve a long-term goal that is both personally meaningful and makes a positive mark on the world."

Your greater purpose is your greatest weapon in conquering your goals. Your goals and action plans will create the path to success. Your why keeps you motivated in your journey. Purpose creates intention in achieving your goals and it makes the pursuit of your goals meaningful. Imagine a life driven, not simply by motivation, but a life driven by purpose. It doesn't just make a bond to your goals; it makes you bound to reach success. Success is imminent!

"If you don't have a purpose, if you don't know what drives you, or what inspires you, you will have no *reason* to improve yourself." -Pedram Zaff

The only way that you'll discover purpose is if you intentionally seek to have a more selfless worldview. You'll never discover a purpose without the selfless why. There are a few pathways to becoming more selfless in your worldview.

How To Become More Selfless

The first path to the selfless worldview is by keeping yourself connected to other people. The more that you can connect with people, see people, feel people, hear people, and love people, the more that you will start to see through selfless eyes. On the flip side, the more disconnected you become, the more selfish you become. And unfortunately, you're not going to build deep relationships through social media or through text. I believe the reason that more than ever before many people are feeling lonely and disconnected is because they are seeking connection through social media. Humans aren't wired to have deep connections through a media source. To be as modern and relevant as possible, no AI boyfriend, girlfriend, or companion will offer the true connection that we need. Put down the phone and be intentional about connecting and spending quality time with the one in front of you. Take the time to have dinner with your loved ones. Take the time to have a true undistracted date with your significant other. Take the time to play with your kids. Take the time to enhance your relationships with others. In doing so, your worldview will become more selfless.

Another path to the selfless worldview is by building a stronger faith. Embracing or discovering a theology of a loving God promotes selflessness as love is selfless. When you connect with people, your purpose is horizontal, but when you connect with your faith, your purpose also becomes vertical. Having faith pulls you into living for God rather than yourself, and you'll began to view your purpose on this earth as a calling. Jeff Bezos once said, "You can have a job, or you can have a career, or you can have a calling. And if you can somehow figure out how to have a calling, you hit the jackpot because that's the big deal." Doing what you feel you are called to do, rather than what you want to do, promotes selflessness.

    While there are many paths to developing a selfless worldview, the last that I believe is worth mentioning is serving and volunteering. Take time to serve other people. Volunteer at a homeless shelter or food pantry. Donating is great, but volunteer at your local charity. Serving and volunteering creates a deeper empathy, love, and care for others and in return gives you a deeper bond to humanity. Giving a homeless man a blanket under a bridge will give you the deeper perspective that someone else needs you. Metaphorically speaking, putting yourself at someone's feet will break any regard for "me." In fact, as an adolescent who struggled with severe depression, serving others through charity became my breakthrough from my severe depression. It put me into a selfless mindset. Serving not only leads to greater connection to people but you'll even receive greater life meaning and fulfillment. While it may seem irrelevant to your success in your fitness goals, your connections are the lifeline in developing a why that is bigger than you.

    We are being conditioned to be selfish, and we are being conditioned to lose connection to others. In a world with greater isolation and a world conditioned to quarantine, there is a fight to maintain true connection. While we are losing our connection with others, we are losing our grasp on our purpose. I believe this lack of purpose is one of the main reasons that more are becoming depressed, feeling hopeless and alone. And why suicide rates are climbing, and fewer are stepping out to do the significant things that they were built to do. It's because we are reaching inward trying to fill a void when we should be reaching outward. The most fulfilling life that you can ever live is to be able to get to a place in your life where your life becomes driven by purpose. If you can break through and live the life of love and selflessness, you will be able to separate yourself from the pack.

  Purpose is what caused me to spend six years of my life traveling from middle schools to high schools to stand in front of audiences as large as 4,000 at a time speaking about how they can overcome destructive behaviors and live a life of freedom. I may have been shaking backstage terrified of stepping on that stage, but it was purpose that made me walk out and grab that mic. It was purpose that drew me into the fitness industry and later the health industry. I wanted to combine my passion for fitness with helping others become successful not just in their fitness journey but in life. It was purpose that caused me to spend four years competing in bodybuilding competitions. It caused me to walk on a stage in nothing more than board shorts to be judged by the thousands of viewers. Beyond my own insecurities and dysmorphias that I was combating was the need to inspire everyone in my audience. It was purpose during my prep that caused me to walk into the gym with my head held high delivering the need to crush my workout. Through it all, I would place at some of the most competitive shows in the U.S. It's now because of purpose that I'm going from being a bodybuilder to a triathlete. If I can completely destroy and transform my physique, if I can go from strength to endurance, and learn to love the cardio that I've always hated, so can you!

  It was purpose that caused me to spend three years writing this book. It caused me to pull off the highway to find the nearest parking lot to write an idea that may have ended up in this book. It was purpose that caused me to spend those multiple times of unplanned three hours of writing in my car in a Tom Thumb parking lot, when I was just going to pick up almond milk from the store. I was never a writer. Growing up, I always hated reading books and I never liked school. But it was purpose that caused me to educate myself on how to write, to start writing, to reading books, and pursuing more certifications and knowledge to write about. The inspiration to start reading and writing this book was because of something bigger than me.

If you can find your purpose behind what you do and live within a selfless worldview, you'll exceed far beyond your expectations. **And there is no soft way to put this, but purpose will give you a responsibility. Someone else is waiting for you to succeed.** In fact, someone is relying on you to succeed. In the pursuit of your goals, it will move you from "I want" to "I must." Imagine if you have a life so driven by a purpose where every goal that you commit to becomes "I must." Failure is no longer an option. Someone's life is going to transform. And someone is going to help someone else transform their life. Be the one.

Final Thoughts

Focusing on the process is about creating systems that keep your transformation constant. To be successful in creating sustainable change is less about the actions you take, and it's more about the systems you create. These actions that I'm referring to are, "I am going to start exercising" and "I'm going to start dieting." These systems that I'm referring to are creating the right environment, meal prepping, scheduling your workouts, hiring the trainer or dietitian, creating affirmations, pursuing greater knowledge, and creating goals and an action plan. Without the proper systems, you will not be able to successfully implement the actions and sustain the actions. The creation of systems is vital to your success.

It's not about making radical changes in a couple areas of your life, but about making small changes in several areas of your life. The number one most important ingredient to your success is in creating a lifestyle that is sustainable. A dramatic transformation doesn't come from a couple of dramatic efforts. A dramatic transformation comes from a dramatic amount of small efforts in several areas of your life. It's the small steps that lead to distance traveled.

Our diet culture has created dirty business. There is no such thing as a one-size-fits-all method to becoming successful in getting results. Fad diets may be effective at delivering temporary results but are completely ineffective at creating a sustainable lifestyle change. A quick-fix approach will never allow you to develop your dream physique.

Transformation starts within the mind. The shift in neural patterns will affect the belief system. The belief system will become the catalyst in the creation of new actions. Those actions, if done routinely, will form new habits. New habits will create new outcomes, and the greatest outcome to be achieved is a changed identity.

The essence of transformation is to be process-focused, not outcome-focused. New outcomes will happen naturally when the process is embraced. When starting your regimen, it is vital to find what you enjoy, whether it's the exercise routine you engage in or the foods you eat. Enjoyment is a must. You'll only grow to the level of those around you, so place yourself in the environment of growth. Discipline is a vital part of the process, especially the disciplines of consistency, self-control, and patience. Only if you embrace the process will you discover the diamond within you.

You will never become a new person with your old mindsets and mentalities. Don't be the victim of your circumstance. Allow your circumstances to make you victorious. Champions become champions because they make the decision to never quit. Be humble enough to keep asking questions. Shut down your pride but embrace the life of confidence. Confidence attracts the greater destiny. See yourself as rich, and it will compel you to invest more into yourself and your own abilities. Don't seek the quick return, pursue the long-term reward. Mistakes are going to happen so don't beat yourself up over imperfection. Constant progress should be the goal.

Based on the most current research and development, there are sure-fire methods to deliver results. Above everything, find the form of exercise that you enjoy, as it will become a regimen that you can sustain. Diet is very complex but luckily we have amazing technologies and resources available to help you identify the right foods for you without having a diet approach. Don't seek after a drug to give you results. Rather, discover the medical issues that are withholding those results. Most medical issues can be corrected through the proper diet and exercise regimen. It is equally important to understand your own body and possible aversions, such as poor hormone health, poor insulin sensitivity, and poor gut health. Becoming aware of such conditions, and how to correct such conditions, can lead to a breakthrough in your journey.

Don't let society condition you, let you condition you. You can master your own life if you can master your environment. Become aware of what's distracting you. If you can eliminate your distractions, you'll be able to be more precise in hitting your goals. Don't sit on the couches of inactivity. Get up and get moving because your solution may not be more cardio but more activity. Keep the kitchen clean and prepare what you need as this will eliminate overindulging. No one else's opinion of you should matter so don't seek validation. Competition is great but comparison is dangerous, especially if we aren't aware of how unrealistic it is to obtain what you are comparing yourself to. Don't hate yourself enough to make changes. Love yourself enough to promote healthy and natural change. Self-love should be your most important relationship goal.

Don't be afraid of the small steps and the small goals. Over time, those small steps will lead to a long distance traveled and the acquisition of your long-term goals. The plans are just as important as the goals themselves. Be creative and make your goals exciting. Motivation and discipline are key factors in being successful in reaching your goals. Remember your why behind the formation of those goals, and you will stay connected to those goals. Seek the life of selflessness to discover your purpose. The purpose makes success inevitable. Success is inevitable, just don't ever quit on your goals.

The last thing that I want to encourage you with is this- At some point within the process, it'll become easier for you. When you keep marching forward, you will eventually look back and realize that it wasn't as hard as you thought it was going to be. The hardest part is when you first start. This is how it is at the beginning of every individual's pursuit of change. If you don't believe me, set your shower to be as cold as it can possibly get, then get in it. Those first 10 seconds are the most challenging. After 10 minutes you'll look back and realize that it wasn't as bad as your originally thought it was going to be. You'll always feel the pain in the beginning because change can be extremely difficult. But you'll adapt to the change and you'll become stronger because of the change. But it's only if you embrace the change and grow through the change, that you'll transform your entire life. Just put one foot forward, and then the next, and don't stop.

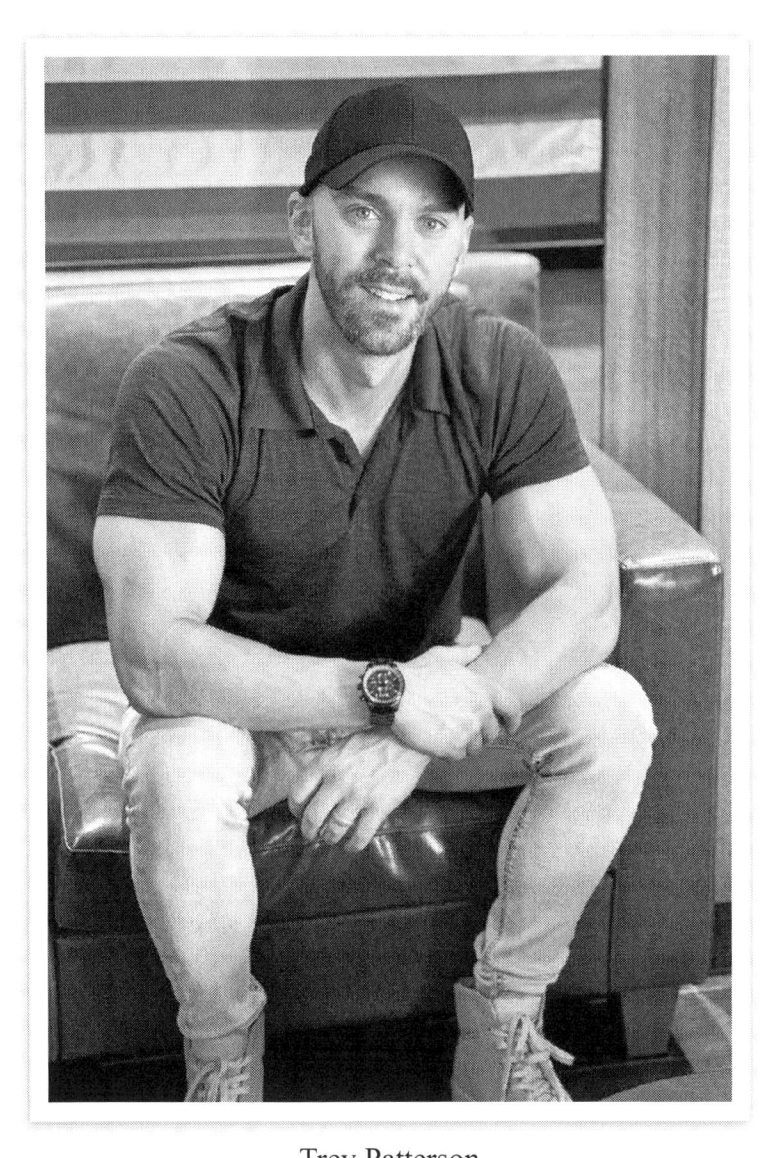

Trey Patterson

B.A. in Communication Theory (Dallas Baptist University)

NASM-CPT (Certified Personal Trainer)

NASM-FNS (Fitness Nutrition Specialist)

NASM-GPTS (Group Personal Training Specialist)

AFPA Certified Health & Wellness Coach

Acknowledgements

I would like to first thank my wife, Monica Patterson, for her continuous belief and support in me. Her unwavering patience and love has allowed me to fully pursue my dreams and my purpose. She endured through all my late nights of writing and was always checking in on me at 1-2 a.m. to make sure I was okay. She is my better half.

I would like to thank every single one of my training clients and friends, especially those whom I wrote about in this book. You are the ones who inspire me day after day and without you and your desire to train with me, there is no me. It's the unknown answers to questions from clients that pushed me into greater knowledge. I have learned because of you. The creation of this book was a team effort.

I would like to thank my mother, Patty Patterson, for her support and her strong belief in me. My mother played a huge role in the creation of this book as she was my first editor and first person to provide valuable feedback. I would also like to thank my father, Mark Patterson, for his support and constant encouragement to me. He was my first coach as he coached every single sport I played as a kid, and whom I always aspired to be like. He taught me how to be a coach.

I would like to thank my two other editors, Nadirah Hill and Robin Hutchins. Nadirah is a journalist who is also a training client of mine, and Robin Hutchins was my favorite communications professor from Dallas Baptist University whom I've kept in touch with for over 10 years. Both Nadirah and Robin have unmatched experience in editing, and this book wouldn't be the book it is without their touch. They have been able to bring this book that has inspired you, to its highest professionalism. I'm beyond grateful for both Robin and Nadirah.

I would like to thank Xhani with 99designs by Vista Print for the amazing book design and his creativity in capturing the image of the book. I would like to thank my publisher Ruth Jones with Let's Go! Press for providing direction in the full execution and completion of this book. There would have been no completion without your hand of help. You have saved my book and have brought The Sustained Fitness Transformation to life.

I would like to thank my several friends that are writers and editors, and thank you for constantly giving me good tips on how to write and how to publish my book. You were such big cheerleaders and supportive throughout my writing journey, and it pushed me to keep going. You know who you are.

I would like to give a special thanks to both Bill Rich and Ryan Binkley. These are two influential individuals in my life that told me that I was going to one day become a writer. It was their words of wisdom that instilled the idea and belief within me that I could write a book.

I would like to thank my Lord and Savior Jesus Christ. Making the decision to follow Christ at the age of 16 was the greatest decision I have ever made, as it truthfully saved my life. It was through discovering Him and building a relationship with Him, that I discovered a greater purpose. This entire book was written through His inspiration and I give Him all the glory. I would not be where I am today, and may not even be alive, if it wasn't for Christ coming into my life.

And last, thank YOU for entrusting me in your sustained fitness transformation journey.

Stay Connected

If you have enjoyed reading The Sustained Fitness Transformation and would like to continue to Train with Trey, please follow me on Instagram and YouTube by scanning the QR codes below. By staying connected, you will receive exclusive content, promo codes for discounted products, and a committed trainer to personally help you achieve greater success.

Instagram:

YouTube:

Citations

Goldstein J, Hagen M, Gold M. Results of a multicenter, double-blind, randomized, parallel-group, placebo-controlled, single-dose study comparing the fixed combination of acetaminophen, acetylsalicylic acid, and caffeine with ibuprofen for acute treatment of patients with severe migraine. Cephalalgia. 2014 Nov;34(13):1070-8. doi: 10.1177/0333102414530527. Epub 2014 Apr 14. PMID: 24733408.

Foundations of Professional Coaching. Siegel, 1999, p.219

Peterson GL, Finnerup NB, Colloca L, Amanzio M, Price DD, Jensen TS, Vase L: The magnitude of nocebo effects in pain: A meta-analysis. Pain 155:1426-1434, 2014.

Nordstoga, A. L., et al .2019. Long-term changes in body weight and physical activity in relation to all-cause and cardiovascular mortality: The HUNT study. International Journal of Behavioral Nutrition and Physical Activity

Fasano A. Leaky gut and autoimmune diseases. Clin. Rev. Allergy Immunol. 2012;42:71–78. doi: 10.1007/s12016-011-8291-x. [PubMed] [CrossRef] [Google Scholar]

Harris MI: Diabetes in America: epidemiology and scope of the problem. Diabetes Care 21 (Suppl. 3):C11–C14, 1998

Divers J, Mayer-Davis EJ, Lawrence JM, et al. Trends in Incidence of Type 1 and Type 2 Diabetes Among Youths— Selected Counties and Indian Reservations, United States, 2002–2015. MMWR Morb Mortal Wkly Rep. 2020 Feb 14;69(6):161–165

Gut microbiota in obesity. Liu BN, Liu XT, Liang ZH, Wang JH. World J Gastroenterol. 2021;27:3837–3850. [PMC free article] [PubMed] [Google Scholar]

Andersson AM, Jensen TK, Juul A, Petersen JH, Jørgensen T, Skakkebaek NE. Secular decline in male testosterone and sex hormone binding globulin serum levels in Danish population surveys. J Clin Endocrinol Metab. 2007 Dec;92(12):4696–705.

McDowell CP, Dishman RK, Hallgren M, MacDonncha C, Herring MP. Associations of physical activity and depression: results from The Irish Longitudinal Study on Ageing. Exp Gerontol. 2018;112:68-75. doi: 10.1016/j.exger.2018.09.004

Global burden of 87 risk factors in 204 countries and territories, 1990–2019: a systematic analysis for the global burden of disease study 2019. Lancet. 2020;396:1223–1249. doi: 10.1016/S0140-6736(20)30752-2

Rachel Krantz-Kent, "Television, capturing America's attention at prime time and beyond," Beyond the Numbers: Special Studies & Research, vol. 7, no. 14 (U.S. Bureau of Labor Statistics, September 2022)

Rachel Krantz-Kent, "Television, capturing America's attention at prime time and beyond," Beyond the Numbers: Special Studies & Research, vol. 7. no. 17 (U.S. Bureau of Labor Statistics, September 2022).

Elgaddal N, Kramarow EA, Reuben C. Physical activity among adults aged 18 and over: United States, 2020. NCHS Data Brief, no 443. Hyattsville, MD: National Center for Health Statistics. 2022. DOI: https://dx.doi.org/10.15620/cdc:120213

Ross C. Brownson, Tegan K. Boehmer, and Douglas A. Luke. DECLINING RATES OF PHYSICAL ACTIVITY IN THE UNITED STATES: What Are the Contributors? Annual Review of Public Health 2005 26:1, 421-443

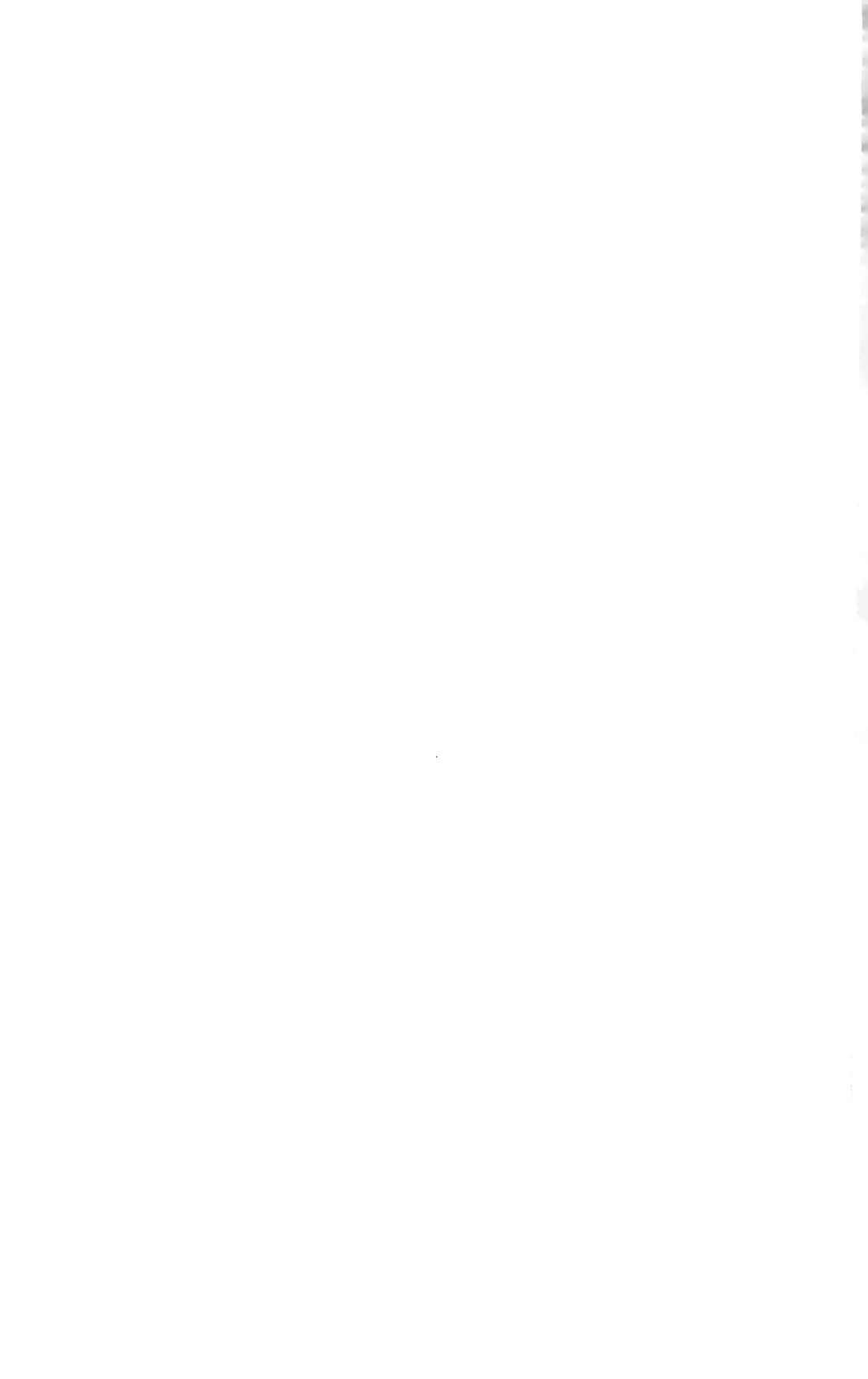

Made in the USA
Columbia, SC
08 April 2025